Praise for other books by Christopher Vasey, N.D.

"If you are plagued by any of the disorders or discomforts ranging from lack of energy to dry skin or from hair loss to arthritis . . . then you will want to read *The Acid-Alkaline Diet for Optimum Health* at your first opportunity to improve your health."

THE MIDWEST BOOK REVIEW

"The only word for Christopher Vasey's *The Naturopathic Way* is brilliant. It is the best overview of the naturopathic approach to healing that I have read."

STEPHEN HARROD BUHNER, AUTHOR OF
THE SECRET TEACHINGS OF PLANTS

"Christopher Vasey has once again written an important book that advances our understanding of health and gives readers a clear approach to detoxification that far surpasses the majority of books in this realm. *Optimal Detox* is a concise, readable, and practical book that puts the power to heal into your own hands. Highly recommended."

MARC DAVID, NUTRITIONAL PSYCHOLOGIST, FOUNDER OF
THE INSTITUTE FOR THE PSYCHOLOGY OF EATING,
AND AUTHOR OF THE SLOW DOWN DIET AND
NOURISHING WISDOM

"Christopher Vasey, N.D., perfectly explains the major importance of a well-balanced biological terrain as well as the need to control the effects of external pollutants and internal pollutants. *Optimal Detox* offers the tools to live a healthier and more youthful life. I highly recommend this book."

YANN ROUGIER, M.D., AUTHOR OF DELTA MEDICINE AND
FOUNDING MEMBER OF THE INSTITUTE FOR APPLIED
NEURONUTRITION AND NEUROSCIENCES

"There is so much to know about cleansing your body of toxins, and somehow Christopher Vasey makes it simple to understand. *Optimal Detox* is a good follow-up to his book *The Acid-Alkaline Diet for Optimum Health*, and both are excellent resource books for professionals and everyday people who simply want to live a healthier life and detoxify from all the toxins in our environment and processed foods."

LOTUS GUIDE MAGAZINE

"*Natural Remedies for Inflammation* contains very valuable information. The author has provided the background of each herb and its dose for a particular health condition. It is easy to read and will serve as a useful source of information for those who are interested in herbal remedies for inflammation."

KEDAR N. PRASAD, PH.D., COAUTHOR OF
FIGHTING CANCER WITH VITAMINS AND ANTIOXIDANTS

"Enthusiastic applause for the combined efforts of Dr. Vasey and the late Mrs. Brandt! Give *The Detox Mono Diet* your full attention, and you will have the foundation for success in self-healing."

CARRIE L'ESPERANCE, AUTHOR OF
THE SEASONAL DETOX DIET AND SOUL BREATHING

"Detoxification is the missing link in Western nutrition, and fasting/juice cleansing is a pure and safe form (over water fasting) of detoxification. Dr. Vasey's very informative book brings light to this vital process through one of the first approaches to cleansing, Johanna Brandt's Grape Cure. There are so many people and so many health conditions that can benefit from this natural health approach found in *The Detox Mono Diet*."

ELSON M. HAAS, M.D., THE DETOX DOC, AUTHOR OF THE
DETOX DIET AND STAYING HEALTHY WITH NUTRITION

Freedom from Constipation

Natural Remedies for Digestive Health

Christopher Vasey, N.D.

Translated by Jon E. Graham

Healing Arts Press
Rochester, Vermont • Toronto, Canada

Healing Arts Press
One Park Street
Rochester, Vermont 05767
www.HealingArtsPress.com

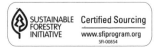

Text stock is SFI certified

Healing Arts Press is a division of Inner Traditions International

Originally published in French under the title *Se libérer de la constipation: Par des moyens naturels*
First U.S. edition published in 2017 by Healing Arts Press

Note to the reader: *This book is intended as an informational guide. The remedies, approaches, and techniques described herein are meant to supplement, and not to be a substitute for, professional medical care or treatment. They should not be used to treat a serious ailment without prior consultation with a qualified health care professional.*

Library of Congress Cataloging-in-Publication Data
Names: Vasey, Christopher. | Graham, Jon E., translator.
Title: Freedom from constipation : natural remedies for digestive health / Christopher Vasey, N.D. ; translated by Jon E. Graham.
Other titles: Se libâerer de la constipation. English | Natural remedies for digestive health
Description: First U.S. edition. | Rochester, Vermont : Healing Arts Press, 2017. | "Originally published in French under the title Se libâerer de la constipation: par des moyens naturels"—T.p. verso. | Includes index.
Identifiers: LCCN 2016018701 (print) | LCCN 2016024496 (e-book) | ISBN 9781620555859 (pbk.) | ISBN 9781620555866 (e-book)
Subjects: LCSH: Constipation. | Digestion.
Classification: LCC RC861 .V3713 2017 (print) | LCC RC861 (e-book) | DDC 616.3/428—dc23
LC record available at https://lccn.loc.gov/2016018701

Printed and bound in the United States by Lake Book Manufacturing, Inc. The text stock is SFI certified. The Sustainable Forestry Initiative® program promotes sustainable forest management.

10 9 8 7 6 5 4 3 2 1

Text design by Virginia Scott Bowman and layout by Priscilla Baker
This book was typeset in Garamond Premier Pro with Helvetica Neue and Gill Sans used as display typefaces

To send correspondence to the author of this book, mail a first-class letter to the author c/o Inner Traditions • Bear & Company, One Park Street, Rochester, VT 05767, and we will forward the communication, or contact the author directly at **www.christophervasey.ch/anglais/home.html**.

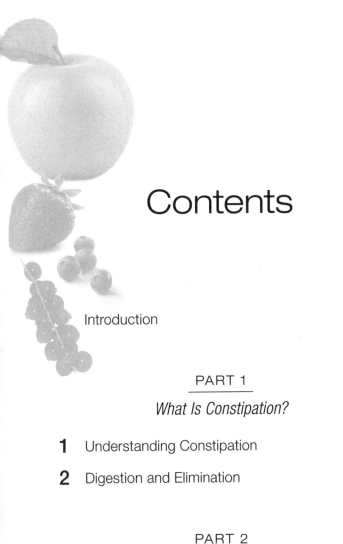

Contents

PART 3

Therapeutic Emptying of the Intestines

Introduction

The purpose of this book is to help the reader discover the likely causes of his or her constipation and the best means to remediate them.

Too many people suffering from constipation are satisfied to take one or another of the large number of remedies—natural or not—that are on the market today. But generally they take these preparations without knowing if the remedies truly correspond to their needs or to the cause of their suffering. Moreover, in the majority of cases these remedies treat the effects—and not the origin—of the problem. Thus, remedies such as laxatives are not really a solution to constipation. They do not attack the root of the problem, which lies in the patient's lifestyle.

Like all organs, the intestines can only function effectively when they are used properly. It is of primary importance to consider the habits of a person suffering from constipation. The person's lifestyle must be examined carefully to discover and correct the causes of her or his constipation.

While the first part of this book explains what constipation is and how the intestines function, the second part of the book—and the most important—focuses on the lifestyle practices that are the causes of this health problem.

There are eight major causes of constipation:

- lack of roughage
- lack of water
- a sluggish liver
- the ingestion of foods or medications that cause constipation
- muscle weakness
- an imbalance of the intestinal flora
- stress
- nutritional deficiencies

Each of these causes is the subject of its own chapter in part 2. Practical suggestions in each chapter for addressing the cause will make it possible to immediately begin relieving the painful condition of constipation. By following the advice provided, readers can support the work of their intestines instead of thwarting them. The intestines will gradually resume their working rhythm, and constipation will vanish.

Part 3 offers several dynamic practices for emptying the intestines: laxatives, purges, and enemas. Here we leave the domain of healthy lifestyle and enter the realm of therapeutic action. This is only an antisymptom therapy, which provides the patient relief by emptying all that is a burden but does not attack the causes that have led to this accumulation. The basic treatment for constipation consists in eliminating its causes by adopting a healthy lifestyle that conforms to the needs of the intestines.

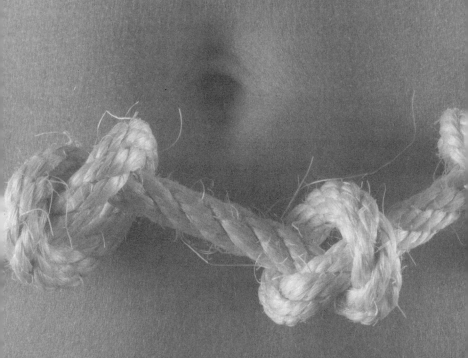

PART 1

What Is Constipation?

1 Understanding Constipation

Constipation is a health disorder characterized by difficulty in obtaining a spontaneous, daily evacuation of a sufficient quantity of the fecal matter contained in the colon.

The root cause of constipation can be related to either the overly slow passage of fecal matter in the intestines or to the dif-

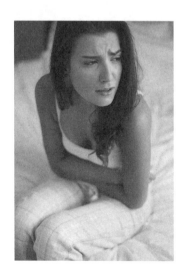

The inability to move fecal matter out of the intestines is the root cause of the painful condition of constipation.

ficulty of expelling the fecal matter once it has reached the end of the colon. In both cases, there is a delay in elimination that leads to the accumulation of matter.

As a condition, constipation presents differently across the wide spectrum of people who suffer its effects. For example, evacuation can be relatively regular but incomplete, or it can be complete but only take place every few days; evacuation can occur on a daily basis but is not spontaneous and requires much exertion; or it may be relatively easy to evacuate the intestines, but the person suffers from several days' stagnation of stools in the colon, and so forth.

THE CRITERIA FOR GOOD INTESTINAL EVACUATION

Many people who live with constipation do not know what it means to have properly functioning intestines. The following criteria describe a normal evacuation of the intestines.

Frequency
Stools should be produced daily. Foods need a period of fifteen to twenty-three hours to be digested and transformed into stools. For many people in the West, whose diets lack adequate fiber and water, this time is significantly increased to fifty-five to ninety-six hours. However, optimal intestinal transit time is fifteen to twenty-three hours.

Speed of Transit
In a period of twenty-three hours, or roughly one day's time, digested food should reach the end of the colon as fecal matter and be ready for evacuation.

Good to Know

The speed of intestinal transit can be measured by eating foods that color the stools, such as beets, which give a red color to the stools, and spinach, which makes them green. The speed of transit can be determined by taking note of the time these foods were ingested and by observing when the red or green stools are evacuated.

Form

The stools have the appearance of a long sausage that coils around itself. It can possibly break into two or three fragments, but not into a large number of pieces.

Consistency

Healthy stools are soft, well molded, and compact. They are also well coated in mucus, which makes it so they do not dirty the anus or the toilet. The use of toilet paper is not necessary.

Manner

The stools are evacuated easily. When the sensation of the need to evacuate is felt and the anal sphincter is relaxed, the stools pass spontaneously and without effort, leaving a sensation of complete emptying.

Color

Normal stools have a slightly brownish yellow color.

Odor

The stools of a person enjoying good health have a slight odor.

THE STOOLS DURING CONSTIPATION

People suffering from constipation will have a completely different experience when evacuating stools from the one just described.

Frequency

Most often, stools are not eliminated on a daily basis but are instead eliminated irregularly, every few days. In the best case, evacuation will occur every two or three days, but it may be every five or six days. In extreme cases of constipation there is only one stool every ten or fifteen days, and evacuation is only produced thanks to laxatives, purgatives, or enemas. In other cases, constipation alternates with short periods of diarrhea, which is the body's way of catching up with its needs for elimination.

Speed of Transit

Stools are formed on a daily basis but are evacuated several days later. For example, the stools evacuated on Friday are not formed from the foods eaten on Thursday but from those consumed on Wednesday or Tuesday. Instead of taking one day to reach the end of the colon, the fecal matter makes this trip in two or three days—or more. Stools formed over several days collect in the intestines, filling a long portion of the colon rather than only its terminal part. The latest arrivals push on those that are ahead of them, which causes the oldest ones near the end of the colon to be evacuated.

Form

The stools are made of several rather short pieces, or broken up into what looks more like goat dung. They can also have a sausage shape but will be hard and rigid.

Consistency

The stools are most often hard and compact, which prevents them from passing easily through the anal sphincter. Their hard consistency is also accompanied by an absence of the lubricating mucus. However, stools caused by constipation can also be pasty and sticky. When this is the case, they are messy.

Manner

The expulsion of stools is laborious. They take longer to come out and require greater effort. Evacuation lacks all the spontaneity that characterizes the movement of bowels in normal circumstances. Evacuation is also not complete—a sensation that something still remains inside will persist.

Bristol Stool Chart

The Bristol stool chart or Bristol stool scale classifies human feces into seven categories. Developed by Dr. Stephen Lewis and Dr. Ken Heaton at the University of Bristol and first published in the *Scandinavian Journal of Gastroenterology* in 1997, the Bristol stool chart is used as a medical aid in determining whether or not a person is constipated.

 Type 1: Separate hard lumps, like nuts (hard to pass)

 Type 2: Sausage shaped but lumpy

 Type 3: Like a sausage but with cracks on its surface

 Type 4: Like a sausage or snake, smooth and soft

 Type 5: Soft blobs with clear-cut edges (passed easily)

 Type 6: Fluffy pieces with ragged edges, a mushy stool

 Type 7: Watery, no solid pieces; entirely liquid

Color

There is no typical stool color during constipation. Their color depends on the foods that have been eaten and the quantity of bile they contain.

Odor

The prolonged stay of the stools in the intestines and the chemical transformations this causes (fermentation and putrefaction) causes them to have a strong, unpleasant odor.

THE HARMFUL EFFECTS OF CONSTIPATION

Constipation creates two kinds of adverse effects. Over the short term it causes feelings of physical and mental discomfort. Over the long term it causes harm to the body's cellular terrain and thus to the person's overall health.

Physical and Mental Discomfort

A person whose intestines have not emptied themselves over a period of several consecutive days will inevitably experience the sensation of feeling "full" and congested. The accumulation of material will give the person the painful impression of a heavy weight in the lower belly, sometimes accompanied by cramps and various pains.

In addition to this unpleasant sensation of being too full, there is also the painful sensation of not being able to empty oneself. The person desperately wishes to empty the intestines in order to feel better, but nothing happens, and the intestines remain blocked. Sometimes the stools begin to move toward the exit, but they cannot move far enough. The need to evacuate is felt at such times, but it is not fulfilled—the stools are on the way but never reach their destination. This feeling is made even more frustrating

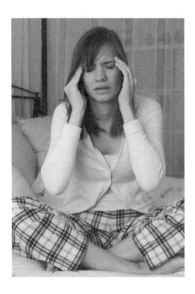

Constipation can lead to mental anguish, including feelings of irritation, frustration, and depression.

by the fact that "pushing" is no help, and that all effort of the will is useless.

This sense of physical discomfort will reverberate on the mental level. A deep feeling of dissatisfaction and frustration will ensue. People suffering from constipation feel irritated. They can become either impatient and aggressive or discouraged and depressed. Their enthusiasm is severely dampened by feeling blocked. They rarely feel at ease. They feel they are not as free and self-confident as they should be. Basically, they find it much harder to feel carefree and full of the joy of living.

Deterioration of the Terrain

The second adverse consequence of constipation is its effect on the physiological cellular terrain. The colon's job is to prepare the stools and then expel them. If the colon's walls were impermeable and did not allow the toxins held in the stools to make their way into the bloodstream and tissues, a delay in the evacuation of the stools, and even the presence of excessive stools, would not be so alarming. The person would just need to be patient, or drain the colon by means of a purge, laxative, or colonic when the situation became intolerable.

Unfortunately, the colon's walls are not impermeable—they allow all kinds of substances to find their way into the bloodstream. The colon's extensive absorption capacity has long been recognized. For example, we know that the pharmaceutical substances contained in suppositories act on the entire body, not only on the colon—their active principles do not remain inside the colon but are absorbed by it. Another example of intestinal absorption can be seen in the results of the nutritional enemas advocated by Dr. Catherine Kousmine to remedy the omega-3 and omega-6 deficiencies of her patients. These enemas consist of a rectal infusion of 60 milliliters (4 tablespoons) of lukewarm cold-pressed sunflower oil before bedtime. The oil is intended to remain in the colon overnight. The bodies of those individuals who are greatly deficient are so greedy for the omegas that they will absorb almost the entire quantity of oil during that time. This can easily be seen the next day, as there will be practically no oil in the stools.

Normally, the mucous membranes of the colon only allow substances useful to the body to cross through them. These substances include nutrients extracted from the food mass, such as water, vitamins, amino acids, and mineral salts. All the other beneficial substances have already been removed during the transit of the food mass through the small intestine. The colon's mucous membranes in fact act like a selective filter. The meshwork of this filter is so small that it only allows small molecules, such as those of nutrients, to pass through. Conversely, they capture the large molecules that are toxins and expel them with the stools, thus prohibiting the toxins from gaining access to the internal terrain of the body.

Constipation will eventually cause damage to this filter. When the stools are stagnant, the toxins remain in constant contact with the colon's mucous membranes. The poisons and toxins contained in the stools, or which develop there from the fermentation and putrefaction of fecal matter, attack the mucous membranes. Once these membranes have been injured, microlesions appear—the filter's mesh has been partially destroyed and larger openings have been formed.

Because of their larger size, these openings offer passage to larger molecules such as toxins. The protective barrier has been broken and toxins are now invading the internal terrain.

THE TERRAIN

Terrain is the word used to describe a concept of major importance in natural medicine. The state of health for the entire body depends on the health of the terrain. (A more extensive study of the terrain can be found in my book *The Naturopathic Way*.) So just what is the terrain, and why does it lead to disease when its condition degenerates?

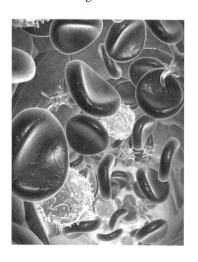

The terrain consists of all the fluids in the body, including those within cells and those in which the cells are bathed.

The terrain is the environment in which the cells of the body live. This is a fluid environment. It is made up of the blood that circulates in the vessels, the extracellular fluid that surrounds the cells, the intracellular fluid that fills the cells, and the lymph that drains toxins out of the tissues.

Together these different fluids represent 70 percent of the body weight, which shows their importance. The cells are fully dependent on these fluids for survival and functioning. They bring the oxygen and nutrients the cells need as well as bringing the toxins produced by the cells to the excretory organs to be eliminated.

Like all living beings, the cells need a healthy environment—a terrain. It so happens that with constipation and the deterioration of the colonic mucous membranes, the toxins that should have harmlessly exited the body are now being absorbed by it. First they enter the bloodstream. When it becomes too thick, the organism pushes these toxins deeper, into the extracellular fluid. Here the toxins collect around the cells, hindering the cells' proper functioning by their presence and injuring the external membrane of the cells by the aggressive substances they contain. Through the pressure exerted by the ongoing arrival of more toxins, those that initially surrounded the cells eventually penetrate to the cells' interiors, disrupting the function of the cells by attacking them.

Blood, the cellular fluids, and lymph are in constant movement. The speed at which they move varies from one fluid to another—it is rapid for the blood and slow for the cellular fluids—but all of them move at one speed or another, and they never stop moving. Consequently, toxins do not only collect in one specific section of the body—they spread throughout the entire organism.

Natural medicine believes that the fundamental cause of disease is the terrain overloaded with toxins.

It is out of an ailing terrain such as this that the majority of our ills develop. Health disorders rarely appear in the absence of accumulated waste. Along with nutritional deficiency, the deterioration of the terrain is the necessary condition for illness to blossom. Deterioration of the terrain is the common feature of all catalogued illnesses, no matter what they are named or how and where they appear.

Toxins are, in effect, the agents that thicken the blood and congest and attack the organs, causing inflammation and lesions, which leads to sclerosis of the tissues. Toxins are also responsible for creating a terrain that is receptive to microbial infections and prone to forming cellular mutations that lead to the development of cancerous tumors.

This notion of illness is not imaginary. It has been verified by clinical studies.

Cardiovascular diseases are characterized by the congestion of the bloodstream and its vessels by toxins of lipid origin, such as cholesterol and saturated fatty acids. The joints of rheumatics are blocked, inflamed, and painful because of toxins—uric acid and others. In respiratory diseases, the waste products that encumber the bronchia, nose, and sinuses are sneezed, coughed, or expectorated out of the body. Pimples, eczema, and hives are all evidence of toxins being eliminated through the skin. In cancer, the cause can be found in carcinogenic substances; in allergies, it is allergens; in celiac disease, it is gluten; in diabetes, it is sugar, and so forth.

Depending on the quantity of wastes and the ability of the patient to eliminate them, the disease will have an acute, chronic, or degenerative nature. These three states are progressive stages that the illness moves through as the clogging of the terrain increases.

Acute diseases are characterized by a violent but brief elimination of toxins, because the strength of the person's defense systems is still high. Chronic illnesses reveal their presence through

ILLNESSES AND TERRAIN DETERIORATION

Illness	Characteristics	Causes
Cardiovascular	Thickened blood, excess cholesterol, fatty deposits in the blood vessels	Excess of saturated fatty acids
Joint	Inflammation, pain	Attacks from toxins
Respiratory	Runny nose, expectorations, coughing	Respiratory tract is overburdened with toxins
Skin	Pimples, eczema, hives	Elimination of aggressive toxins through the skin
Cancer	Development of tumors	Cellular mutations caused by toxins
Allergic	Inflammatory reactions	Allergens
Celiac	Digestive disorders and diarrhea	Gluten
Diabetes	Numerous functional disorders, those caused by lesions	Excess sugar in the blood and tissues

less violent eliminations that get established over time and are repeated at more or less regular intervals. The person's strength has diminished and is not sufficient to eliminate all the excess toxins in one go, as is the case with acute disorders. In the beginning, chronic diseases are functional, but over time the toxins begin attacking the tissues themselves, creating lesions. Degenerative diseases are characterized by a greatly weakened defense system that has been worn down from having to cope with a terrain that has become incredibly congested. The body can no longer defend itself, or at best can only make a weakened effort. The toxins disrupt the functioning and the very structure of the organs, as is the case in cancer, multiple sclerosis, autoimmune diseases, and evolving chronic polyarthritis, to name a few.

THE STAGES OF DISEASE

Illness	Elimination	Vitality	Duration
Acute	Strong	Strong	Short
Chronic	Average	Diminished	Long and recurring
Degenerative	Weak or absent	Weak	Permanent

CONSTIPATION'S INFLUENCE ON THE TERRAIN

Any eliminatory weakness of the colon inevitably leads to auto-intoxication. As stools stagnate, the toxins contained in fecal matter are partially absorbed by the body. In this way the body poisons itself with its own toxins, something that would not have happened if the stools had been evacuated normally.

The colon is not the only excretory or eliminatory organ at the body's disposal, though. There are several others. The liver eliminates wastes in bile, the kidneys expel waste in urine, the skin in sweat and sebum, and the lungs in the gas exhaled. (For more on this see my books *Optimal Detox* and *The Detox Mono Diet.*) Poor functioning of these organs also leads to the congestion of the terrain and the creation of numerous diseases. Nonetheless, the colon remains one of the most important excretory organs, not only because of the volume of the wastes it eliminates from the body, but also because it is the organ that eliminates the toxins filtered out by another excretory organ—the liver.

Because of the deteriorated condition of the terrain it causes, constipation should not be considered as a localized affliction without any connection or influence on the rest of the body. The repercussions of this disease affect the entire body by means of

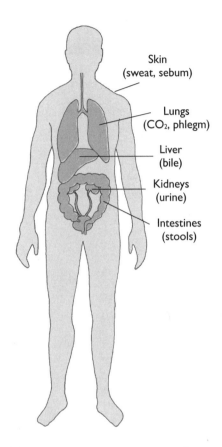

Skin
(sweat, sebum)

Lungs
(CO_2, phlegm)

Liver
(bile)

Kidneys
(urine)

Intestines
(stools)

The five excretory organs
are the pathways by which
we eliminate toxins

the terrain. A person affected by constipation consequently is rarely suffering from this illness alone. Over time, because of the accumulation of toxins in the tissues, other health disorders begin to appear. However, the connection between this toxin accumulation and constipation is rarely made, because a terrain that is deteriorating takes some time to show on the "surface" in the form of illnesses.

In the past, doctors always asked their patients about how their intestines were functioning. An important part of the therapy they implemented consisted of emptying the colon of the matter that was burdening it and stimulating its work in order to guarantee regular and complete eliminations of stools. Enemas, purges, and laxatives that were recommended so often in the past are often ridiculed today. They are considered to be a vestige of an archaic and ineffective medicine.

It so happens that in these standard practices the doctors of yesterday were attacking the root of the illness: the overload of the terrain by toxins. They went to work on the profound nature of illnesses; hence the surprising success they enjoyed in treating numerous health disorders. Of course, therapy should not be restricted to emptying of the colon, but not taking it into account is a serious mistake. This unfortunately is more and more the case today, as people have lost the knowledge of the importance of the terrain and good eliminations. Treatment is concentrated on the consequences of toxin overload, not on the causes of the overload. Medications cause disease symptoms to disappear, but not the toxins saturating the cellular terrain and creating the symptoms. The terrain remains congested by toxins, and as they continue to accumulate, illnesses appear, becoming increasingly serious over time. Fighting constipation therefore requires not only getting rid of an unpleasant ailment; it also means working on the terrain and on the health of the whole body. Many people have been able to see this for themselves: the treatment that rids them of constipation also heals them of other disorders.

WHAT TO DO ABOUT CONSTIPATION?

The first reaction of a person confronted by constipation is to try to empty the intestines as soon as possible. Consequently most people have no hesitation about using radical means to get rid of what is weighing them down. Purges are the most expeditious means to achieving this end. (See chapter 11 for a discussion of purges.) Several hours after taking a purgative, the entire contents of the intestine are expelled out of the body. The effect of enemas is even quicker but less thorough. They affect the terminal end of the colon, whereas purges empty the colon in its entirety. Another means of draining the intestines is laxatives. They function much like purges, but in a softer and gentler way.

These different therapies have been known since the dawn of time. A five-thousand-year-old Egyptian papyrus mentions them. Even animals will resort to them. Ailing cats eat couch grass to purge themselves; elephants ingest muddy clay for the same purpose. Using these methods to drain the intestines therefore seems fully legitimate. However, in reality this is not the case. These therapies only empty the intestines; they do not restore the intestines to their proper functioning. They are useful for bringing quick relief, but their effect does not last.

Moreover, they do not act on the causes of constipation. In fact, a person is not constipated because he or she failed to take laxatives; constipation happens for an entirely different reason. The stools the body eliminates easily are those that have been prepared properly. This preparation takes place along the entire length of the digestive tract. The famous naturopath P. V. Marchesseau (1911–1994) rightly claimed: "Good digestions make good stools"—which is to say, stools that can be evacuated with no problem.

When you are suffering from constipation, it is therefore important not to concentrate solely on the colon and confine yourself to only seeking the means to empty it. To the contrary, it is imperative to expand your vision of things and consider the entire digestive tract.

In the next chapter I present the various stages of digestion, up to evacuation of the stools, to show that, indeed, good digestions make good stools.

2 Digestion and Elimination

The foods we eat cannot be used as they are by the body. Their volume is too large and their chemical structure too complex for the cells. Consequently, the foods we ingest must be prepared by the body to be usable. This preparation takes place during digestion.

During the digestive process, the food we take in is divided into smaller and smaller particles. Once that has been achieved, the nutrients—vitamins, minerals, amino acids, and so forth—now isolated from the framework of the food are absorbed by the intestinal walls, then transported by the bloodstream into the cells. All that remains—the non-utilized parts of the food—is evacuated.

However, remains are not eliminated in that state. Rather, through the digestive process the non-utilized food matter is given the shape and consistency necessary for an easy evacuation from the colon.

> In the process of digestion, nutrients are extracted from the food we eat and are delivered to the cells. The non-utilized food matter is given the shape and consistency necessary for easy evacuation from the colon.

Transformations therefore take place at different stages of the digestive tract. These transformations are primarily digestive in purpose as food matter moves to and through the small intestine, but from the colon on the digestive process is entirely focused on the elimination of the stools.

THE MOUTH

The teeth tear apart the food, cutting it into smaller morsels; then, by crushing these morsels repeatedly, they pulverize the food. The mechanical grinding caused by mastication is accompanied by secretions of saliva (approximately 1 liter per day) by the salivary glands. With the water it contains, saliva softens the food particles and encourages them to dissolve. Saliva also contains digestive juices that attack the very structure of foods. It consists primarily of ptyalin, which breaks down carbohydrates (starch). The long molecular chains are divided into shorter segments.

The blend formed by crushed food and saliva is known as the alimentary bolus, or chyme. Due to its liquid nature, it can easily move downward from the mouth to the esophagus.

THE ESOPHAGUS

The esophagus—the tube that leads into the stomach—begins just behind the mouth. It measures almost 10 inches in length. Its walls contain rings of muscle. By contracting one after the other, the muscles create a wave of contractions. This peristaltic movement pushes the food mass downward. Through this action and the liquid nature of the alimentary bolus, the foods we swallow find their way into the stomach. The need to drink that we may sometimes feel while eating happens when the swallowed alimentary bolus is not fluid enough. The food mass has trouble advancing and stagnates in the esophagus. The water that we drink

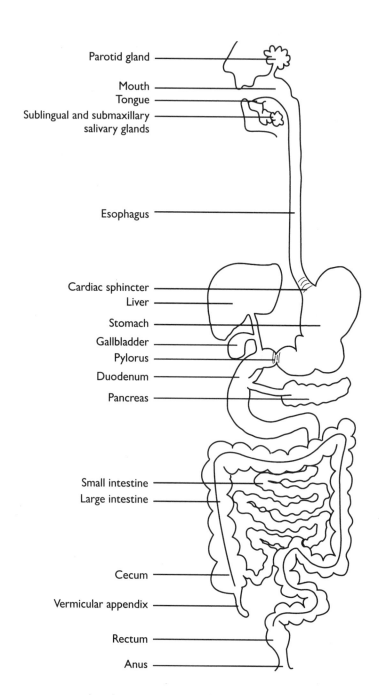

Parotid gland

Mouth

Tongue

Sublingual and submaxillary salivary glands

Esophagus

Cardiac sphincter

Liver

Stomach

Gallbladder

Pylorus

Duodenum

Pancreas

Small intestine

Large intestine

Cecum

Vermicular appendix

Rectum

Anus

The digestive tract and its glands

moistens the alimentary bolus and helps transport it down into the stomach.

The entry of the alimentary bolus into the stomach is controlled by the lower esophageal sphincter at the end of the esophagus. This ring-like muscle closes the exit of the esophagus when it contracts. This closing makes it possible to delay food from entering the stomach when necessary and also prevents the contents of the stomach from coming back up, as in the condition known as acid reflux.

THE STOMACH

The stomach is a pouch approximately 10 inches long, 4¾ inches wide, and 4 inches from front to back. Its walls are extendable, so much so that the volume of the stomach increases when it is full—for example, after a heavy meal—but shrinks when it is empty. The stomach is equipped with powerful muscles that allow it to contract. These kneading movements mix the alimentary bolus, dividing the food particles into even smaller pieces. This peristaltic movement also ensures that the alimentary bolus is evenly saturated with the digestive juices secreted by the gastric mucous membrane.

On average, the stomach produces 1 liter of gastric juices a day. Their primary role is the digestion of proteins. Gastric juices are extremely acidic; they have a pH of 2. This acidity has a highly corrosive effect on the hard particles contained in the alimentary bolus, but also on the walls of the stomach. The walls protect themselves by secreting a mucus that prevents the gastric juices from reaching them.

While foods only remain for a period of seconds in the mouth, they will stay in the stomach for one to three hours. The exit point of the stomach is also equipped with a sphincter: the pylorus.

Normally it is closed. It opens selectively to allow water and the parts of the alimentary bolus that have been properly transformed to pass through. The others are kept in the stomach to be kneaded and attacked further by the enzymes of the gastric juices. When all the transformations that can take place at this level have been completed, the pylorus opens and the alimentary bolus moves into the top of the small intestine.

THE SMALL INTESTINE

The small intestine begins with the duodenum, which is shaped like the letter C. This area receives some extremely important secretions for digestive transformations: those of the liver and pancreas. The liver secretions act on fats, while the pancreatic secretions act on proteins, carbohydrates, and fats. These digestive juices blend with the alimentary bolus and act on it during its entire passage through the small intestine.

The small intestine is a tube approximately 5 meters (16 feet) long and 3 centimeters in diameter. While the duodenum is fixed

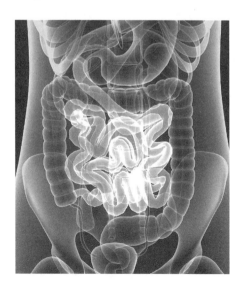

The liver and pancreas secrete their digestive juices into the small intestine.

in place, the rest of the small intestine is not. It is capable of moving a little in the space that holds it inside the abdomen. Given its length, and the small space at its disposal, the small intestine does not descend in a straight line but instead forms numerous coils.

The alimentary bolus advances through this long, sinuous tube thanks to the contractions of the ring-like muscles of the walls of the small intestine. By contracting one after another in succession, they create peristaltic waves that push the alimentary bolus forward. The remaining particles that are too large are attacked by digestive juices released by the small intestine itself (3 liters a day).

After a period of four to eight hours, the nutrients contained in the alimentary bolus are ready to be absorbed by the body. This takes place at the level of the intestinal villi, threadlike projections that cover the wall of the small intestine. The nutrients travel through the wall to enter the bloodstream, which transports them to the liver to be distributed to the entire body.

Assimilation of nutrients takes place primarily in the bottom half of the small intestine. Water is assimilated here as well. Some of that water is the liquid we drink, but most is contributed by the digestive juices. In fact, 7 liters of digestive secretions reach the intestines: 1 liter of saliva, 1 liter of gastric juice, 1 liter of bile, 0.75 liter of pancreatic juices, and 3 liters of intestinal juices. This substantial amount of fluid is not eliminated with the stools; it is mostly reabsorbed and reutilized by the body. Normally, the body has enough liquid at its disposal to easily produce these great quantities of digestive juices. When this is not the case, which is to say when a person does not drink enough and his body is dehydrated, intense thirst will be felt when he starts to eat. It is in fact during meals that these juices are secreted, and therefore it is at this time that the body begins drawing fluids from the tissues to manufacture the digestive juices.

THE DIGESTIVE SECRETIONS

Organ	Digestive Juice	Volume
Salivary glands	Saliva	I liter
Stomach	Gastric juices	I liter
Liver	Bile	I liter
Pancreas	Pancreatic juices	0.75 liter
Intestines	Intestinal juices	3 liters

Once the nutrients have been extracted from the alimentary bolus, the food mass does not disappear. It remains present and contains all the substances that could not be digested. This is primarily cellulose—the hard, resistant fibers of vegetables that escape the enzymatic activity of the human body's digestive secretions—as well as undigested food particles (proteins, fats, and so forth). Added to this are a mass of dead cells from the intestinal walls, which are regenerating continuously.

Once the alimentary bolus reaches the lower end of the small intestine, it makes its way into the colon.

THE COLON

The colon plays no role in the digestion of the alimentary bolus, which may explain why the walls of the colon are not covered with villi, like the small intestines. The colon's role consists of transforming the residues of the digestive process into stools. Of course, this work of transformation will free up some additional nutrients that will be absorbed by the walls of the colon. Nonetheless, the colon's primary role remains the preparation of stools—the fecal matter to be eliminated. This is the reason that, once the partially digested food mass reaches the colon, it is no longer called the alimentary bolus but is instead referred to as the fecal bolus.

The colon's role consists of transforming the residues
of digestion into stools.

The clear-cut difference between the role played by the small
intestine and that played by the colon is evidenced by the fact of
the sphincter that separates them—the ileocecal valve. This valve
only opens to allow the alimentary bolus to enter the colon. The
rest of the time it remains carefully closed to prevent the flow of
fecal matter into the small intestine. The intestinal compartment
responsible for nutrition and the one responsible for wastes are
therefore quite distinct.

The colon is the continuation of the small intestine. At
3 to 5 centimeters, the colon's diameter is larger than that of the
small intestine (3 centimeters for the small intestine). It is because
of this wider diameter that the colon is described as the large
intestine—as opposed to the intestine with a smaller diameter,
the small intestine.

The colon measures 1.5 meters in length. It travels along the
periphery of the abdomen and forms a kind of frame, in the center of which is the small intestine. It is made up of three principal parts: the ascending colon begins in the lower part of the
right flank and climbs vertically to the level of the liver. There
the colon takes a turn and horizontally traverses the abdomen to
the left side of the body—hence its name, the transverse colon.
(In reality the passage of the transverse colon is not truly horizontal, as it bends somewhat downward toward the navel and then
climbs back up.) Its orientation allows the contents of the colon
to be kept longer at this level for the purpose of transforming
them before turning them over to the descending colon—which,
because it is vertical, allows the contents to quickly find their way
to the exit. The descending colon begins at the top left flank,

then descends vertically a ways before bending toward the center of the abdomen. This bend is known as the sigmoid colon. The end portion of the colon consists of the rectum or rectal ampulla and a short tube leading to the anus. This tube is equipped with a sphincter for controlling evacuations.

As it plays no digestive role, the colon does not secrete any digestive juices. The transformations that occur in this region of the body—the preparation of stools—are made thanks to the intestinal flora. This flora consists of a multitude of tiny organisms, or bacteria, that specialize in the decomposition of the various materials present in the colon.

Ten to twelve hours are needed for the colon to form stools out of digested food matter. This is a long time and is revealing of the scope of labor necessary for their preparation. But this preparation is an essential step to ensure that the stools are able to be expelled easily. This evacuation occurs thanks to the combined efforts of the peristaltic muscles of the colon and the contraction of the abdominal muscles.

DURATION OF THE STAGES OF DIGESTION

Stomach	1 to 3 hours
Small intestine	4 to 8 hours
Colon	10 to 12 hours
TOTAL	15 to 23 hours

Various points about digestive tract function discussed here will be referenced in the next part of this book, as they play a key role in the battle against constipation.

PART 2

Attaining and Maintaining Intestinal Health

3 Roughage and Constipation

The foods we eat descend into the stomach, then transit though the small intestine and, lastly, through the colon. This entire pathway is more than 7 meters long. Food is not capable of moving through this course without the aid of an external force. This force is a function of the intestines themselves—the process known as intestinal peristalsis.

INTESTINAL PERISTALSIS

The word *peristalsis,* from the Greek, means "to envelop, to compress." When they contract, the walls of the intestines envelop and compress the matter they contain. Intestinal contractions do not take place simultaneously along the entire length of the intestines but instead occur in discrete portions of the intestines at a given time. The process of peristalsis begins at the top of the small intestine; the enveloping and compressing movement then travels gradually through the length of the intestines until the motion reaches the farthermost parts at the end of the colon. In this way, progressing along the length of the intestines, the suc-

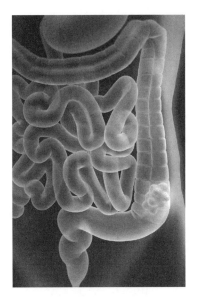

By contracting, the intestinal walls envelop the substances they are holding and compress them.

cessive compressions create a wave of intestinal wall contractions. The phenomenon repeats and gives birth to what is called the "peristaltic movement" of the intestines.

> By progressing along the length of the intestines, the successive contractions of the intestinal muscles create peristaltic movement.

The process takes place thanks to two kinds of muscles arranged in overlying layers in the intestinal walls. The outer layer is formed of longitudinal muscles, which means that the fibers are oriented in the direction of the length of the intestines. The inner layer includes muscles whose fibers are called "circular" because they surround the intestines; these are perpendicular to the longitudinal muscles.

The advance of food matter in the intestines results from the harmonious collaboration of these two kinds of muscles. The longitudinal muscles are responsible for advancing the material through the intestines. But to ensure that this progression only follows the right path, which is to say toward the lower end of the intestines, the circular muscles also play an important role. They contract after the substances have passed, to prevent food matter from moving backward, while relaxing in front of the food matter to give it free passage.

This activity of the intestinal muscles takes place progressively through the entire length of the intestine in a repeated manner. This is how one peristaltic wave follows another, gradually moving the contents of the intestines toward the end of the colon.

Like any other muscle, intestinal muscles only work when they have received an impulse. This impulse is given to them when, under the pressure of the intestinal content, both the longitudinal and circular muscles can no longer maintain their resting shape. The stretching out of the intestinal fibers through the introduction of food matter sends the signals to the muscles that they should contract. This only happens when the intestine is quite full. When the intestines are empty or holding only a small amount of substance, no signal is given—the intestinal muscles remain in a state of rest, no peristaltic movement occurs, and the food matter remains in place.

THE IMPORTANCE OF ROUGHAGE

What gives volume to intestinal content are materials that are of a certain mass and that, for this reason, take up a certain amount of space in the intestines. They therefore also must possess a structure that does not disintegrate during digestion. These materials that are endowed with a certain consistency or solidity are fibers that come from foods of plant origin, such as fruits, vegetables, whole grains, oleaginous fruits such as nuts and olives, and beans.

These include, for example, the fiber of leeks and beet greens, the veins of the leaves of salad greens, the husks of cereal grains, and the skin and seeds of fruit.

> **The fibers from plant-based foods give bulk to intestinal content.**

Generally speaking, plant fibers do not break down under the effects of digestive enzymes. Instead, they retain their shape and structure, forming roughage, the filler material the intestines need to function properly.

The solid nature of these fibers balance and oppose the softness and absence of structure of other materials making up the intestinal content. Cheese, eggs, and meat contain no fiber. During the digestive process, these foods are easily broken down into their constituent elements. Foods of animal origin consequently do not create a solid mass that fills the inside of the intestines but instead create a soft, malleable mass that flows but does not fill the intestines. It does not cause the intestinal walls to stretch and therefore does not trigger intestinal peristalsis.

The roughage the intestines require to function properly is formed solely of fibers of plant origin. These fibers play no nutritional role as the body cannot digest and absorb them. The role they play in elimination, however, is fundamental. Without plant fibers the intestines could not rid themselves of the material they hold.

The sources of roughage are:

- fresh fruits, dry fruits, and oleaginous fruits such as nuts and olives
- vegetables
- beans
- grains

It is important to note that the grains I am referring to here are whole grains. In the process of refining cereal grains to make white flour and white rice, the outer layers of the grain (the bran) are removed. But it is precisely in these surface layers of grains that the fibers can be found. By ridding grains of these layers, we are also depriving our intestines. So when we eat refined grains, such as white bread, white pasta, and white rice, we are denying ourselves one of the primary sources of roughage that nature has given us for the proper functioning of our intestines.

THE TWO KINDS OF PLANT FIBER

Plant fiber can be divided into two groups, each with distinct characteristics, that act in their own way on the intestines. These two kinds of fiber are present in all foods of plant origin but exist in varying proportion depending on the food.

- *Water-soluble fibers:* These fibers are primarily composed of pectin and mucilage. These substances combine easily with water and produce a soft, viscous gel. Water-soluble fibers also swell when they are moistened; thus their increase in volume is quite high, doubling and even quadrupling in size—and in some cases their volume can be multiplied ten times.

- *Fibers that are not water soluble:* These fibers are hard and firm. A good example of this kind of fiber is the cellulose of wheat bran. At contact with water, cellulose will become permeated with liquid, but in contrast to soluble fiber, it will not swell in size. The volume of these kinds of fibers therefore does not increase once in the intestinal tract.

THE FIBERS

Fibers	Examples	Origin	Characteristics
Soluble	Pectin mucilage	Fruits	Swells and becomes jellified
	Mucilage	Flaxseed	Swells and becomes jellified
Insoluble	Cellulose	Grains	Becomes permeated with liquid

All plant fibers give bulk and consistency to the stools simply by their presence. But in the case of water-soluble fibers, the volume obtained is higher than when originally ingested. Furthermore, thanks to the great capacity for holding water that this type of fiber possesses, these fibers stay moist as they move through the intestines. This is helpful to know for those people whose constipation is caused not only by a lack of fiber, but also because their stools are too dry.

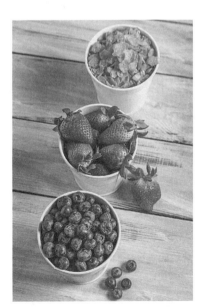

Plant-based foods such as fruits and cereals are high in water-soluble fiber.

The average requirement for fiber is estimated at about 30 grams a day. This daily quantity is generally not achieved in the modern Western diet. Today's daily fiber intake is more likely to be around 12 grams. The current everyday diet in the West is in fact characterized by the predominance of foods of animal origin—such as meat, fish, cheese, and eggs—foods that lack fiber. The modern diet also includes many grain products, such as bread, crackers, and pasta, but since these are prepared from refined grains they no longer contain the valuable fiber from the original plant. Furthermore, the average diet is often poor in raw vegetables, fruits, and beans, the very foods that possess the fibers intended by nature to ensure the effective functioning of our intestines.

A fundamental cause of constipation today is this lack of roughage. An important means of treating constipation consequently consists in giving the intestines the fibers they require.

THE FIBER CONTENT OF VARIOUS FOOD GROUPS

Fiber content varies from one food to the next. Some foods are quite rich in fiber while others possess far less. While emphasis must be placed on the high-fiber-content foods when addressing constipation, this does not mean that other plant-based foods should be neglected. The fibers we need are not meant to be supplied by only one or two foods out of all those that exist. We must also include in the diet the many foods whose fiber content is lower, but that together with fiber-rich foods can add up to providing the necessary total.

Furthermore, some foods are rich in fiber but cannot be eaten in great quantity, whereas foods that contain less fiber can be eaten in larger amounts. For example, almonds contain up to

14.5 grams of fiber per 100 grams, whereas carrots only contain 3 grams. It is difficult, however, to eat 50 grams of almonds, while it is entirely possible to eat 250 grams of carrots. The quantity of fiber consumed is identical.

The following tables show the overall fiber content, both water soluble and not, of various foods. They are classified according to the food group to which they belong. The fiber content of the actual food will vary in accordance with its origin, variety, maturity, and the meteorological conditions in which the food is grown (a hot, dry summer or a wet and cool one). These variations result in fiber content being listed variously by different authors. I have used figures from the French food-composition databank Ciqual in these tables.

The various food groups will be presented, with the foods in each group ranked according to fiber content.

Grains

Cereal grains such as wheat, rye, and rice are rich in fiber due to the protective husk that surrounds each kernel. This husk is made from hard cellulose, which is not soluble in water. It is therefore not broken down during digestion and remains almost entirely available for use as roughage. This husk is removed in the process of producing white flour and white rice.

Good to Know

The fiber content of grains in the table on page 38 is only applicable to unrefined, whole grains. The more refined the grain, the smaller its fiber content. While complete grain flour contains 11 grams of fiber, whole grain flour contains 8.5 grams, and white flour only 3 grams. Unrefined brown rice contains 6 grams, while white rice contains 1 gram.

FIBER CONTENT OF GRAINS
(per 100 grams)

Barley	17 g
Rye	15 g
Wheat	12 g
Oats	11 g
Spelt	11 g
Buckwheat	10 g
Millet	9 g
Corn	7 g
Quinoa	7 g
Rice	6 g
By-products	
Wheat bran	43 g
Oat bran	15 g
Cereal flake blends	5–25 g

Vegetables

The majority of vegetables have a fiber content in the range of 1 to 3 percent of their weight in grams. Whether the edible part of the vegetable is its leaf, stem, root, or fruit does not matter a great deal. The vegetables with the highest fiber content are not that much higher than the others. These high-fiber-content vegetables include chicory, kohlrabi, dandelion, brussels sprouts, and green beans, each of which contains 4 grams of fiber per 100 grams, and artichokes, parsnips, and green peas, which contain 5 grams.

Although their fiber content is not that high, the advantage of vegetables is that they can be eaten in large quantities. Consumed as cooked vegetables, in salads, as raw crudités, sautéed, or baked, the quantity of vegetables consumed in a meal can easily exceed 250 grams. Cooking will soften fibers, but that does not change the quantity made available to the intestines.

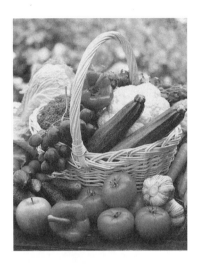

Vegetables have a fairly low fiber content, but they can be eaten in large quantities, which helps to meet the body's daily need for fiber.

Good to Know

To ensure an ample intake of fiber, whenever possible do not peel vegetables or remove the veins from their leaves, as it is precisely in these parts of the plant that most of the fiber will be found.

FIBER CONTENT OF VEGETABLES
(per 100 grams)

Artichoke	5 g
Green peas	5 g
Parsnip	5 g
Brussels sprouts	4 g
Chicory	4 g
Dandelion	4 g
Green beans	4 g
Kohlrabi	4 g
Beet	3 g
Broccoli	3 g
Carrot	3 g

FIBER CONTENT OF VEGETABLES (cont'd)

Eggplant	3 g
Escarole	3 g
Fennel	3 g
Salsify	3 g
Shallot	3 g
Snow pea	3 g
Sweet potato	3 g
Cabbage	2–3 g
Arugula	2 g
Asparagus	2 g
Cauliflower	2 g
Celery	2 g
Leek	2 g
Onion	2 g
Potato	2 g
Radish	2 g
Spinach	2 g
Sweet corn	2 g
Swiss chard	2 g
Turnip	2 g
Lettuce	1–2 g
Pepper	1–2 g
Cucumber	1 g
Pumpkin	1 g
Tomato	1 g
Zucchini	1 g

Fresh Fruits

The fiber content of fresh fruits generally runs from 1 to 2 percent of the fruit's weight. Some fruits—such as pears, figs, kiwis, persimmons, and bananas—are slightly higher at 3 to 4 percent. Fruits belonging to the berry family, including raspberries and red currants, have even more fiber. Passion fruit holds a place all its own with a fiber content of 10.5 percent. Like vegetables, fruits do not contain a record fiber content, but the fact that they are easy to eat in large quantities make them a good source of fiber.

Good to Know

To receive the maximum benefit from the fiber contained in fruits, they should be eaten with their skins on and with their seeds, as appropriate (as with grapes).

FIBER CONTENT OF FRUITS
(per 100 grams)

Passionfruit	10.5 g
Raspberry	7 g
Blackberry	5 g
Persimmon	4 g
Red currant	4 g
Banana	3 g
Fig	3 g
Kiwi	3 g
Pear	3 g
Orange	2–3 g
Apple	2 g
Apricot	2 g
Blueberry	2 g
Cherry	2 g
Clementine	2 g
Mandarin orange	2 g
Mango	2 g
Peach	2 g
Strawberry	2 g
Grape	1 g
Grapefruit	1 g
Pineapple	1 g
Plum	1 g

Dried Fruits

The fiber content of dried fruits is higher than that of fresh fruits. With the water they contained removed, the concentration of their remaining elements is automatically increased.

Good to Know

When dried, bananas figure among the fruits that are highest in fiber, but other substances they contain make bananas a cause of constipation.

FIBER CONTENT OF DRIED FRUITS
(per 100 grams)

Banana	10 g
Fig	10 g
Pear	8 g
Date	7–8 g
Apricot	7 g
Prune	7 g
Cranberry	5 g
Raisins	4–7 g
Apple	3 g

Oleaginous Foods

The oleaginous foods include all the fruits and seeds that have a high oil content, such as nuts and olives.

In addition to their high oil content, these foods are generally rich in cellulose—from 3 to 27 percent of their weight in grams. They can therefore supply a generous intake of fiber. These concentrated, caloric foods require much digestive effort; consequently they can only be eaten in smaller quantities. However, when eaten regularly in small amounts, they contribute to the total intake of fiber necessary for good intestinal function.

FIBER CONTENT OF OLEAGINOUS FOODS
(per 100 grams)

Flaxseed	27 g
Almonds	12–14.5 g
Hazelnuts	10 g
Pistachio	10 g
Coconut	9 g
Sunflower seeds	9 g
Brazil nut	8 g
Avocado	7 g
Walnut	7 g
Pumpkin seeds	6 g
Cashews	3 g
Olives	3 g

Beans and Other Legumes

Leguminous plants—a category that includes lentils, peas, peanuts, and beans—are plants whose fruit is a seedpod. These seeds

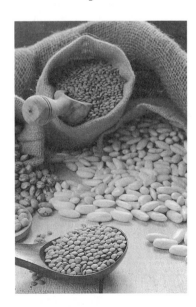

While leguminous plants are high in fiber, they can be difficult to digest.

are characterized by a very high concentration of proteins, but also of fibers. This is the reason they are harder to digest—their reputation for causing flatulence is well deserved.

The laborious digestion that legumes cause creates a great amount of gas in the intestines, and this is why their consumption is not very popular these days. Still, while there is no valid reason for people who customarily eat them—and because they eat them regularly, digest them well—not to continue to eat them, others would probably be well advised to only consume legumes as an occasional supplement. The fiber content of legumes, in the form of raw and dried seeds, is between 9 grams and 31 grams.

FIBER CONTENT OF LEGUMINOUS FOODS
(per 100 grams)

Lentils	31 g
Split peas	24 g
Chickpeas	17 g
Black beans	16 g
Kidney beans	15 g
White beans	15 g
Soybeans*	10 g
Peanuts	9 g

*Tofu, which is prepared from soybeans, contains no fiber.

PRACTICAL SOLUTIONS

DIETARY REFORM FOR CONSTIPATION CAUSED BY LACK OF ROUGHAGE

When lack of roughage is the cause of constipation, your diet is inadequate and must be remedied. Food choices must be examined and changed if you want to see any improvement.

Below I discuss the food choice errors that are leading to con-

stipation. I will explain what is at work in each of these errors and
how to correct the situation.

Predominance of Foods of Animal Origin

The Error

Meals are composed mainly of foods of animal origin, such as
meat, fish, cheese, desserts made from dairy products, and eggs.
These foods are devoid of fiber, as shown by the table below.

FIBER CONTENT OF FOODS OF ANIMAL ORIGIN
(per 100 grams)

Cheese	0 g
Custard	0 g
Eggs	0 g
Fish	0 g
Meat	0 g
Poultry	0 g
Seafood	0 g
Yogurt	0 g

The predominance of these foods in the daily diet can take
two forms:

- the foods are consumed in much greater quantity than
  other foods
- the foods appear more often in meals than the others

Their quantity and the frequency with which they appear in
the daily diet ensure that animal products clearly surpass plant-
based foods, the only food source that contains fiber.

The meal of a person eating this way will primarily consist of

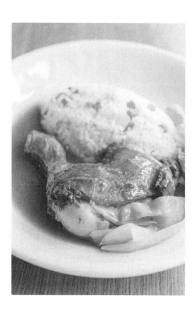

A typical meal composed primarily of animal products

a large piece of meat accompanied by a little starch (rice or pasta, often refined and therefore practically devoid of fiber) and a small portion of raw or cooked vegetables. The meal will end with a dairy-based dessert such as custard, a cream tart, or ice cream. The bread eaten during the meal is quite often white bread, which is equally lacking in fiber. A meal such as this is roughly two-thirds food without fiber and one-third with fiber.

The Solution

This error can be corrected by reversing the proportion of the food groups. Instead of only eating one-third of the meal in the form of vegetables, increase that amount to two-thirds and reduce the foods of animal origin to one-third.

Concretely, this means accompanying the protein (which should not be eliminated if you wish to maintain a balanced diet) with a generous portion of green salad or crudités (raw carrots, fennel, and radishes, for example) as well as cooked vegetables. The starches (pasta, rice, and so forth) should be whole grain, which is to say not refined, so that you can benefit from the fibers they also contain.

When a person is not used to eating raw vegetables, I recommend a gradual reintroduction into the diet. The intestines of a person who has never or rarely eaten raw vegetables will not be accustomed to the hard fibers they contain. Vegetables can sometimes irritate the intestinal walls when they are eaten in too large a quantity, causing cramps, spasms, and bloating.

It may also be necessary to reeducate the person's taste buds. Many people who never eat raw vegetables will have the impression that they have no taste. A readjustment period is often required for the person to again perceive all the variety and subtlety of flavors in vegetables. Over time, the pleasure of eating vegetables returns, making it possible to consume the quantities necessary to provide the intestines with enough fiber.

Primary Consumption of Refined Grains

The Error

Some people's diet consists primarily of refined grains, such as white bread, pasta, and white rice. Such a diet is almost completely devoid of fiber.

Every day we eat numerous foods made from grains. Grains form our principal supply of fibers, as their fiber content is high and they are foods we eat in large quantities (several hundred grams a day, on average). If practically all of the grain-based foods that are chosen are the refined variety, the person's fiber intake will be practically nonexistent.

The Solution

The error of eating a diet based primarily in refined foods can only be corrected by switching to whole grains. In concrete terms, this can be achieved by eating:

- whole grains such as rice, barley, and buckwheat
- whole grain bread
- whole grain pasta
- whole grain cereal flakes
- whole grain crackers
- whole grain granola bars

It is important to make this transition slowly so that the introduction of whole grains can be supported physically and psychologically. Physically, it is necessary to make this transition gradually in order for the intestines to become slowly habituated to the fiber it is now receiving in larger quantity, and that is also harder in texture than what the intestines have heretofore been digesting.

> Grains form our primary supply of roughage,
> as their fiber content is high.

Psychologically, the need for a transition period has to do with the fact that often the obstacle to the introduction of complete grains is the mistaken idea that they do not taste good or are less pleasing than refined grains. For example, many people believe that whole grain rice does not have a good taste or that it is less pleasing than white rice. The same thing is often said about whole grain bread. However, these are natural foods. When eaten as nature intended, they cannot help but be pleasant to taste and take into our bodies.

Good to Know

Experience shows that, after a short transitional period, the majority of people who make this switch consider whole grains and the products made from them, such as bread or pasta, to be more flavorful than refined grains.

There are different varieties of whole grain rice, breads, and pastas. Flavors and textures vary from one kind to the next. Discovering which varieties you like can be an adventure and a joy.

Another erroneous idea is that whole grain rice retains its hard texture even after cooking. In reality, cooked whole grain rice is tender. If it is hard, it has simply not been cooked long enough.

That said, people should not go to the other extreme and banish all refined foods from their diets. Eating a piece of cake made from refined flour from time to time will not lead to adverse health consequences.

A simple, pleasant way to begin increasing your consumption of grains is to start eating a blend of whole grain cereal flakes for breakfast. It is best to stay away from the sugary cereals, whether whole grain or refined.

Insufficient Consumption of Cooked Vegetables

The Error

One reason that some people eat few or no cooked vegetables is that they do not consider them an important part of the meal. They prefer more concentrated foods, such as meats and starches. Another reason often mentioned is that cooked vegetables have no taste. Whatever the reason, people who eat few or no cooked vegetables deprive themselves of an important supply of fiber.

The Solution

Vegetables are not secondary foods—they should be one of the basic foods of our diet. Their rich supply of vitamins, minerals, and trace elements means they should be eaten regularly and in generous quantities. Doing this ensures not only that they will become a valuable and flavorful element of our meals, but that they will also supply a lot of fiber to the diet.

When vegetables truly have no taste it is most often because they have been overcooked, often in too much water. To receive their full benefits it is necessary to ensure that vegetables are cooked in very little water—they should be either braised or steamed. Organically grown vegetables most often have more flavor than those grown by industrial agriculture methods.

Good to Know

An easy means for increasing the intake of fiber is to make a vegetable-based soup and add a small quantity of whole grains such as barley, oats, or quinoa to the soup pot.

The Extremely Limited Consumption of Raw Vegetables

The Error

Some people consider raw vegetables such as salad greens, lettuce, carrots, radishes, celery, kohlrabi, beets, fennel, and so forth to be minor foods used to make side dishes that are served either as appetizers or decorations. Given the scant importance these people grant raw vegetables, they hardly ever eat them, if at all.

The Solution

Reintroducing raw vegetables to the diet is easy once we begin looking at them as the important foods that they are. They are

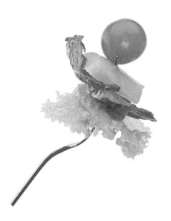

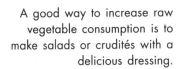

A good way to increase raw vegetable consumption is to make salads or crudités with a delicious dressing.

important because of their wealth of nutrients as well as their high fiber content. Raw vegetables or crudités are often not appreciated because of the salad dressing used to season them. It may be too vinegary or have a taste that people are not used to or do not like. Care should be taken to make a dressing that will be to each person's taste.

Introduce raw vegetables to the diet gradually to allow the intestines time to become accustomed (or reaccustomed) to them. Serving raw vegetables at the beginning or end of a meal is quite normal in many cuisines. The quantities should be generous—a large plate rather than a small bowl.

The Limited Consumption of Fresh Fruits

The Error

Some people eat very little fresh fruit—they only rarely consume it as a dessert or as a snack between meals. Most often this is a habit that is motivated by no precise and well-thought-out reason. Some people abstain from including fruit in their diets with the claim that fruits are not good for them because they ferment in their intestines and cause bloating. Others, who don't want to put on weight, are afraid of fruit's sugar content.

The Solution

The fact that fresh fruits, just like raw vegetables, are one of our best sources of vitamins is great motivation for increasing their consumption. By eating more fresh fruit you will at the same time be increasing the intake of a fiber-rich food. Care should be taken to select the ripest fruits, which will also have the best flavor. In fact, the riper the fruit the sweeter it will be. Some people find fruit easier to eat when it is made into a salad or mixed with yogurt, cottage cheese, fromage blanc, or a bit of cream. Fruit's sugar is natural and therefore easy to metabolize. If you eat fruit, you may also be less tempted to eat foods rich in white sugar, with which one easily puts on weight. Furthermore, the sugar content of fruits is much lower than that of processed sweets.

Good to Know

The bloating or gas that fruit causes is produced primarily when fruits are eaten at the same time as other foods, especially if the meal includes grains. This problem can be easily resolved by eating fruit by itself, as a snack between meals.

One Exception

It is in the best interests of people who are incapable of completely metabolizing the acids of fruits to be very cautious in their consumption of fruits in order to avoid making their bodies overly acidic. (For more on this see my book *The Acid-Alkaline Diet for Optimum Health.*) A person who is extremely sensitive might have to abstain from fruits completely, at least for a certain period of time. Their vitamin needs can then be met by eating larger portions of raw vegetables, or by eating dried fruits, which are generally low in acids. People whose sensitivities are not so acute should try to only eat very ripe fruits (they are less acidic) and only in small quantities (such as eating half of a sweet apple, for example).

Absence of Dried Fruits

The Error

Eating dried fruits such as dates, figs, and prunes is another means of getting fruit into your diet. Yet for many people these fruits are entirely absent from the diet, and thus they do not receive the benefits of the fibers that these foods contain.

The Solution

Dry fruits are rich in sugar, and the sweet taste makes them a pleasure to eat. They are also energy producers. They are therefore a beneficial replacement for snacks such as chocolate, crackers, and pastries, whose white sugar content is generally high and whose fiber content is low or nonexistent.

Good to Know

Dried fruits contain very little acid. They can therefore advantageously replace fresh fruits in the diet of people who are sensitive to fruit acids.

Absence of Oleaginous Foods

The Error

The importance of oleaginous foods is often underestimated. Many people never eat them, or when they do it is unintentional, such as when the oleaginous foods are part of a prepared dish. Almonds, hazelnuts, pumpkin seeds, olives—all of the oleaginous foods have exceptional nutritional qualities, and their fiber content is not negligible.

The Solution

Oleaginous foods can be eaten as snacks, individually or mixing several different kinds at the same time. Or they can be mixed with dried fruits or added to crudités and salads.

Absence of Leguminous Foods

The Error

The importance of beans and other leguminous foods is only a problem for those who customarily ate them and then suddenly stopped. If the foods they are now eating as a replacement for the beans are not as rich in fiber, they will have to contend with a lack of roughage.

The Solution

These people should take precautions to ensure they maintain a certain intake of leguminous foods, since their intestines are accustomed to them, or make sure the legumes are replaced by foods that contain an equally high fiber content, such as whole grains.

When beans and leguminous foods have not been part of your customary diet, you should not go full bore introducing them. In fact, for beans and legumes to act favorably on the intestines, you need to eat them regularly. The drawbacks they create (indigestion, gas, and bloating) are often greater than the advantages they bring (fiber).

FIBER-RICH FOOD REMEDIES

Often, reforming the diet is enough to restore normal intestinal function. Sometimes, though, this is not the case, especially at the beginning of a therapeutic regimen. The intestines have become lazy; they may also be weakened or dilated. Consequently, until they have regenerated they need a much higher than usual quantity of fiber in order to function properly.

In situations such as this, it becomes necessary to resort to foods characterized by a high fiber content or in which the quality of fiber is especially effective. The food remedies that are most often used—because they are the most effective—are bran, psyllium, and flaxseeds.

These foods do not replace a diet already rich in fiber, but they do complete it. A change in diet is thus essential in all cases. This does not mean taking these complements all at once, but using the one that is necessary for your own specific situation. Most often, it requires experimenting with several in order to find the one that is most appropriate.

Bran

The bran of cereal grains such as wheat, oats, and rice is the outer envelope of the grain. The purpose of this husk is to protect the grain from outside attacks, especially contact with water. The husk needs to be hard and resistant. It has these qualities thanks to the many firm, rigid fibers of which it is made. These fibers are made up of long chains of glucose—more than 10,000 units linked together. Since our digestive juices cannot break them down into smaller particles, these fibers, called cellulose, remain unchanged in the intestines and help give volume to the alimentary bolus and stools. They are all the more effective at achieving this outcome because bran is exceptionally rich in fiber, at around 43 grams per 100 grams of wheat bran (15 grams for oat bran). It should be mentioned here that bran does not swell at contact with water, unlike psyllium and flaxseed, two other fiber-rich foods that we will look at next.

Bran is generally defined as the residue from the milling of grain. It is not a residue, though, unless you are seeking to make

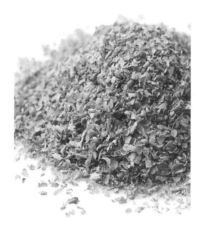

Wheat bran is produced in the milling of the whole grain.

white flour. In the process of making white flour the surface layers of the grain are thrown away after milling; what is left is primarily the starch of the central part of the grain, which, thanks to its light color, permits the making of white bread. While the white bread may be a more attractive color to some, it is devoid of fiber. Consequently, it contributes nothing to the formation of well-molded stools.

In the past, bread was made from whole flour. The bran was not eliminated but was instead considered an integral part of the flour—the bran gives a deep brown color to the bread. The rich fiber content of this bread automatically contributed to maintaining a healthy intestinal transit. The making of complete flour and whole grain breads popular today aims at again offering consumers real bread. This bread is not only rich in fiber but also in vitamins, minerals, and amino acids, as these nutrients, like bran, are found in the surface layers of the grain.

What I've just said here about flour and bread applies to all the other products made out of white flour: pasta, crackers, cakes, pastry—you name it. The other cereal grains can also be rid of their cellulose-rich outer envelopes. When they are, the white rice, pearled barley, and other processed foods that are produced are just as fiber deficient as white bread.

Form

Bran looks like cereal flakes but is thinner and has a hard, fibrous consistency. It is generally sold in bulk in health food stores. Bran can also be obtained in the form of tablets to be swallowed with water.

As a general rule, it is specifically wheat bran that is used to fight constipation. However, over the last few years oat bran has become increasingly popular for this purpose as well. According to some studies, oat bran is more effective than wheat bran at carrying the cholesterol in the alimentary bolus out of the body, making it more helpful for fighting high cholesterol. This property is useful, but it plays no role in combating constipation. For this reason, any kind of bran (wheat, oats, rice) can be used, as it is the roughage itself that interests us.

Good to Know

Whenever possible it is best to eat organic bran. Since bran forms part of the outer husk of grains, the bran can contain traces of the chemicals used to grow the crop if it is not farmed organically.

Taste

Bran has practically no taste and no odor. It has to be chewed in order to get a faint flavor of straw or bread.

Dosage

The best dosage is highly individualized. Start with a teaspoon of bran a day, then gradually increase the daily dose by an additional teaspoon every day. For some people, the dosage may increase to several tablespoons a day.

How to Take It

When taking a small dose of bran it can simply be swallowed with water. However, the fibrous consistency of bran makes it not very pleasant to eat alone in larger dosages. When taking more than a teaspoon or so, it is best to mix bran into another food such as yogurt, soup, sauces, porridge, mashed potatoes, pureed vegetables, or dessert.

Precautions

Because of its rough nature, bran can have an irritating effect on sensitive intestines. In this case it would be better to use psyllium or flaxseed, both gentler alternatives.

When to Take It

As bran is most often taken with food, it is consumed at meal times. Two or three smaller portions are preferable to eating a large portion at one meal. But to simplify things, and if your body can tolerate it, it is possible to take one large dose.

Good to Know

In addition to its laxative effect, bran also contributes to reducing high cholesterol. Its fibers imprison the cholesterol present in the alimentary bolus, preventing it from being absorbed by the body.

Psyllium

Plants of the plantain family share the characteristic of producing extremely mucilaginous seeds. The most often-used variety is the Indian plantain (*Plantago ovata*), also known as ispaghula.

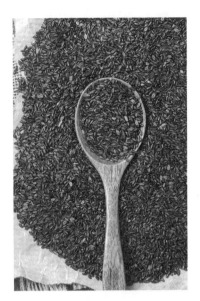

The tiny Indian plantain seed, or ispaghula, is the basis for psyllium.

The term *psyllium* refers to the coarse powder obtained from the Indian plantain seeds or their husk. *Psyllium* comes from the Greek and means "flea." It takes 500 of these seeds, as tiny as fleas, to equal 1 gram in weight.

The Indian plantain seed and its husk contain as much as 30 percent mucilage, which represents a very high fiber content. Furthermore, this mucilage is extremely hydrophilic, which means that its capacity to retain water is very high. At contact with water, psyllium in fact increases to more than ten times in size. This rate of swelling is exceptional. In comparison, the rate of swelling of flaxseeds, which is already quite high, is 5 percent.

The soft, moist, voluminous gel that it forms takes up a large space in the intestine and stimulates peristalsis.

Form

Psyllium can be bought in the form of flakes, powder, seeds, and gel caps.

Taste

The mild taste of psyllium makes it easy to use.

Dosage

The quantity of psyllium needed to stimulate the intestines will be different for each person. Everyone must determine the right dosage for her- or himself by starting with small amounts and gradually increasing the dosage. When the desired results are obtained, you should maintain that dose.

Example of this progression: 1 teaspoon a day for three days, then 2 teaspoons a day for three days. Then 3 teaspoons a day and so on until the right dosage is found.

How to Take It

- Powder: Blend psyllium with water in a drinking glass and swallow it right away. Rinse the glass with more water to get the remaining deposits, and drink that.
- Grains: If you are using whole seeds instead of powder, they need to be steeped in water for several hours before swallowing. This will prevent the grains from collecting at one spot in the digestive tract and swelling there in a compact mass.

Precautions

To avoid all risk of obstruction, it is recommended that you drink a large glass of water (3 deciliters) after taking psyllium in order to spread it out evenly throughout the digestive tract.

When to Take It

Psyllium should be taken before or between meals.

If it needs to be taken several times throughout the day, the dosages should be repeated over the course of the day. When one dose is sufficient, psyllium should be taken in the evening, which generally leads to positive results the following morning.

Good to Know

Psyllium also has the effect of reducing hunger. Taken shortly before a meal, it will swell and fill the stomach. When eating a meal, the feeling of satiation will appear more quickly and you will eat less.

Flax (**Linum usitatissimum**)

Flax is a plant with pretty blue flowers that has been cultivated for centuries because its stems produce strong fibers that are ideal for weaving into cloth. However, it is not these fibers that are used to fight constipation, but the fibers provided by the flaxseeds.

Each mature flax flower will produce a capsule containing approximately a dozen seeds 2 to 3 millimeters long. The seeds have a long, stretched shape; they are shiny, deep brown, and smooth. They consist of 27 percent highly hydrophilic fibers, which is to say they attract and retain water. When flaxseeds come in contact with water they grow five times larger. The viscous, moist gel this produces amply fills the intestine and thereby has a stimulating effect on peristalsis. They also have another effect. Flaxseeds are composed of 46 percent oil, the lubricating properties of which facilitate the progression of the stools.

Flaxseeds are commonly used to fight against constipation. They increase stool volume by making stools moist and by lubricating them.

Form

Flaxseeds are used either whole or slightly crushed. The flax flour that is used to prepare poultices is not at all suitable for the purpose of stimulating the intestines. It quickly turns rancid and should not be ingested.

Taste

When they are swallowed whole, flaxseeds have no taste or odor. When they are chewed, they have a pleasant flavor slightly comparable to hazelnuts.

Dosage

Dosage will differ in accordance with individual needs. Start with 1 even tablespoon, then gradually increase the dosage until it is as high as 2 to 3 tablespoons a day. Some people may require an even higher dosage.

How to Take It

- Add flaxseeds to a little water, and drink the whole concoction. To be sure the flaxseeds swell sufficiently, drink another large glass of water (3 deciliters) immediately after.
- Flaxseeds can also be added to various food dishes: yogurt, salad dressing, fruit salad, applesauce, fruit compote, muesli, and granola, to name a few.
- Instead of swallowing the flaxseeds you can also chew them, which permits their flavor to be enjoyed. It is good to divvy up the times that flaxseeds are taken during the day in order not to have to chew too many of these seeds at one time. By chewing them you can see how the contact of the seeds with fluid (saliva, in this case) produces a gelatinous mass.

Precautions

After each dose of flaxseeds, drink a large glass of water to get the maximum benefit out of the seeds' swelling potential and to help them descend deeply into the digestive tract.

When to Take It

Flaxseeds can be taken at mealtime or between meals; it is up to the person to decide.

Good to Know

Flaxseeds are very rich in omega-3 oils. Flaxseed oil is 54 percent omega-3.

---

4 Water and Constipation

In the preceding chapter we saw how important a generous intake of roughage is for proper intestinal function. Another indispensable element in this regard is water. (For an in-depth discussion on the many health benefits of water, see my book *The Water Prescription*.) Water plays a major role in the formation of stools, and in proportions that are quite substantial. In fact, stools are composed of only 25 percent dry matter (roughage); the remaining 75 percent of stool composition is water.

The purpose for the presence of water in the stools is to make them soft and moist so they will be able to advance easily in the intestines. When there is a lack of water, stools are hard and dry, and their movement through the colon is difficult.

The influence of a liquid's fluidity on the speed of its flow is well known. A stream flows more easily and rapidly when its water is pure, not muddy. This same principle holds true on the organic level as well. Extremely liquid stools, such as those produced during diarrhea, are eliminated easily (albeit uncomfortably). But when stools are hard and dry, as is the case with constipation, they are very difficult to evacuate.

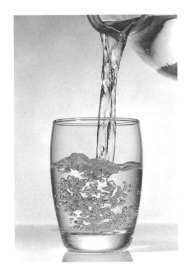

Water is a major component in the formation of healthy stools.

As we have discussed, the length of the intestines is approximately 6.5 meters: 5 meters in length for the small intestine and 1.5 meters for the colon. This represents a long route for material substances to travel. This tube does not go down in a straight line from the stomach to the anus. Instead, it follows a very twisty course that hinders the advance of substances. And while it includes descending vertical sections in which the substances can easily travel, some sections of the intestines are horizontal while others, such as the ascending colon, are vertical and travel in an upward direction. Intestinal peristalsis makes it possible to overcome these obstacles to movement, but only if the stools have the right consistency.

The body precisely monitors this process to ensure that the stools have an optimum water content: just moist enough to avoid constipation, but not too moist so as to avoid the risk of diarrhea.

As stated, on average stools are composed of 75 percent water. They are still considered normal if this rate falls to 70 percent or rises to 85 percent. But falling below or exceeding these limits by even 2 or 3 percentage points will immediately create constipation or diarrhea.

> Many people are constipated because their
> stools lack water.

Generally, the daily stools eliminated by healthy people weigh between 150 and 200 grams. Seventy-five percent of this weight is represented by water, corresponding to 1 to 2 deciliters. The body should have no difficulty providing this fairly small amount of water. And yet, many people suffer constipation because their stools are lacking water. To understand how this is possible, we need to look at how liquid intake is managed by the body.

THE BODY'S WATER NEEDS

The quantity of water the body needs every day is 2.5 liters. This figure has been determined by measuring the volume of liquid that the body eliminates on a daily basis.

The kidneys are responsible for eliminating the most substantial volumes of water. On average, the human being excretes 1.5 liters of urine. The skin sweats out 0.5 liter of liquid every day. The lungs also eliminate a certain quantity of water in the form of water vapor that is expelled with each exhale; this invisible liquid represents 0.4 liter of water every day. The intestines are the final path for water to be eliminated. As we have seen, our stools contain 1 to 2 deciliters of water.

In total, these water excretions represent 2.5 liters of water. Therefore this same amount of water must be restored to the body if we want it to function normally. This intake is provided by the beverages we drink and by the foods we eat.

The absorption of liquids by the body takes place primarily in the intestines. Contrary to the stomach, which only has a digestive function, the intestines also possess an assimilatory function. They are the organs that absorb the nutritious substances extracted from food and from water.

Of the two intestines, the small intestine has greater absorption capabilities. More than 90 percent of the water provided to the body is absorbed by the small intestine. Its capacities are so strong that even if large amounts of water are drunk in a short period of time, they do not go directly into the colon but are instead assimilated by the small intestine.

As the alimentary bolus reaches the colon, the water that accompanies the food mass can be as much as 1 liter. This volume gradually diminishes as stools are formed. The walls of the colon gradually absorb the fluid, leaving just enough to give the stools the consistency necessary to be easily evacuated. Thanks to the body's ability to regulate the moisture content of the stools, we go from 1 liter at the start of the colon down to the 1 to 2 deciliters water content that compose the stools when they are exited from the body.

What I have just described is the normal process for stool formation and evacuation in regard to water. For dehydrated people, the process is different.

A dehydrated person is not replacing the 2.5 liters of fluid that she excretes daily. The reasons for this could be that the person's diet does not include enough water-rich foods or that the person is not drinking enough over the course of the day. Let's look at these two factors.

All foods contain water, but the amount varies from one food to another. The water supplied by foods should ideally be around 1 liter, with the rest provided by drinks. The foods that have the highest water content are:

Vegetables	approximately 90%
Fruits	approximately 85%

The foods that are poor in water are:

Pasta	approximately 61%
Meat	approximately 60%
Soft cheeses	approximately 53%
Bread	approximately 35%
Hard cheeses	approximately 34%
Jam	approximately 30%
Butter	approximately 17%
Cereal flakes	approximately 12%
Crackers	approximately 7%
Chocolate	approximately 1%
Chips	approximately 0%

When foods that are poor in water content are predominant in a person's diet, as is often the case today, the water intake provided by food is insufficient. This is the case with all people who eat few fruits or vegetables.

According to a number of studies, the daily consumption of beverages should be between 2 and 2.5 liters. Factoring in the 1 liter of fluid from food that is provided by a healthy diet, this amount of fluid intake is higher than the 1.5 liters of fluid that would normally be required to balance the average daily excretion of 2.5 liters of water. What is the reason for this suggested volume of daily fluid intake?

There are four reasons for this, all of which are connected with our modern lifestyle.

- Salt consumption today is three times higher than what our bodies actually need. Salt increases the body's water needs.
- There is a general tendency today to overeat. The more we eat, the more water our bodies need to dilute and eliminate toxins.

- It is also generally agreed that modern life is increasingly stressful. Stress causes perspiration, and thus a loss of water.
- The aeration of our homes and offices by mechanical systems (air conditioning, forced hot air heating, and so forth) have a tendency to dry out the body.

For all these reasons it is recommended that a person drink from 2 to 2.5 liters of water a day. In practice, many people do not drink this much, and some don't even consume half this amount. They believe they are drinking enough because, as they say, they never feel thirsty. In fact, their bodies *are* suffering from a lack of water, but their alarm signals are defective. When people do not react to the sensation of thirst, this signal atrophies and eventually stops alerting the need for water.

DEHYDRATION AND CONSTIPATION

Insufficient intake of water, whether from food or beverages or both, will lead to dehydration of the tissues. This must be avoided at all costs, because when dehydration becomes extreme it leads to all kinds of metabolic disruptions. These will be minor initially but become increasingly serious as the dehydration becomes more pronounced and extensive with time. The principal reason for these disruptions is that a lack of water in the tissues interrupts the body's enzymatic activity—the enzymes, which are responsible for all the biochemical transformations that take place in the body—can no longer perform their work properly.

To avoid tissue dehydration, the body uses every means at its disposal to get enough water. As it is incapable of generating more water on its own, these actions will primarily be focused on the body managing the water it does have differently. It will take water from one organ where its presence is not so important and give it to an organ that has a greater need for it. By transferring water this way, the body is able to limit the damage caused by dehydration, at least for the short term.

It so happens that one organ in which a water deficit does not jeopardize the body's survival is the colon. The water the colon holds is only used to eliminate the stools. This is an important function, but not as important as the functions performed by vital organs such as the heart, brain, or liver. This is why, although the colon needs water to prepare stools, the body will take water from the colon in the event of dehydration. This water will be absorbed by the body through the walls of the colon. Transported by the bloodstream, the water will make its way to another part of the body. When water is removed from the colon in this way day after day, the eventual result is chronic drying and hardening of the stools—or, in other words, constipation.

PRACTICAL SOLUTIONS

WHAT TO DO WHEN CONSTIPATION IS CAUSED BY A LACK OF WATER

There are two ways to remedy the problem of stools that are too dry.

The first consists of drinking more water to increase daily consumption. The intended purpose is not to get more water directly to the colon. This will not happen, as the bulk of the water a person ingests will be absorbed by the small intestine. The real purpose of this strategy is to address the dehydration of the entire body, a dehydration that compels your body to take water from the colon. In fact, the problem is not that the colon is lacking water, as it only needs 1 to 2 deciliters to perform its tasks, but that the water it does contain is taken away by the dehydrated body.

The second way to fight against dehydration of the stools

consists of using foods or remedies that attract and retain water in the intestines.

Let's take a look at these two ways to moisten stools.

Drink More

How Much

By drinking 2.5 liters of water a day you ensure good hydration of the body. When this amount of water is taken in on a daily basis, the body will no longer need to make excessive subtractions of water from the colon, which causes the stools to become drier. The volume of ingested water can even be increased to 3 or 3.5 liters for several weeks by people who have been severely dehydrated. People who lead extremely stressful lives or perspire a great deal should drink a quantity adapted to their personal situation.

What to Drink

Water is the primary drink that nature offers us, and it should be the beverage to which we give top priority. This can be water

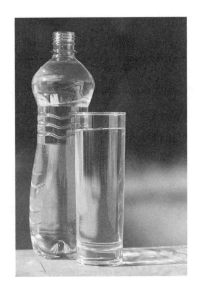

One way to insure adequate daily water intake is to prepare bottles of beverages to meet your daily need and then drink from them throughout the day.

from the tap if it is of good quality. If it is not, bottled spring water or mineral water is a good choice, but don't drink water that is too mineralized. The water you drink can be flat or sparkling, depending on your taste, but it is more natural to drink flat water.

Equally recommended are unsweetened infusions of plants such as mint, verbena, and linden. Fruit juices or vegetable juices—pure or diluted with water—are also among recommended beverages.

Some beverages—such as tea, coffee, cocoa, and sweet commercial sodas—should be avoided, as they do not possess the same hydrating virtues of water. Although they supply the body with liquid, the body does not get much benefit from it. The water these beverages offer the body is almost entirely used to eliminate the poisons, such as caffeine, or the refined sugars that these drinks contain. Furthermore, the diuretic nature of some of these beverages (most notably of coffee) causes the body to lose more water than they bring to it. For obvious reasons, alcoholic drinks are not recommended.

How to Drink

In practice, it is important to drink outside of mealtimes, especially if large amounts of water are required to remedy constipation. This will avoid diluting the digestive juices, a situation that disrupts digestion. It is also preferable to drink in quantities of 3 deciliters at a time seven or eight times a day, rather than taking tiny swallows every few minutes.

Begin your day by drinking one or two large glasses of water upon waking. The water can be cold or warm, according to your preference. Continue with two more glasses over the course of the morning, and two or three in the afternoon. In the evening, after dinner, it is good to have more water, but perhaps in smaller amounts so as to avoid having to get up at night to use the bathroom.

People who customarily drink less than 1 liter a day should not start drinking 2.5 to 3 liters of water daily right away. Instead, gradually increase water intake over the course of one or two weeks to get up to the 2 to 3 liters the body needs. Do not be guided by the sensation of thirst—the signal for which can become defective over time with a lack of water intake—but instead focus on the goal of drinking 2.5 to 3 liters a day. Over time the sensation of thirst will be restored, and you will be able to rely on it again to adjust your liquid intake.

Attract Water into the Colon

Drawing water into the colon from the tissues, with the goal of hydrating overly dry stools, is made possible by the process of osmosis.

Osmosis is a phenomenon that occurs when two fluids of varying density are separated by a permeable membrane. A movement of water (osmotic transfer) takes place from the center of the less concentrated milieu—the one that has the least amount of solid substances in suspension—toward the most concentrated, until the densities of the two liquids are equalized. This transfer takes place because the more concentrated fluid exerts a stronger pressure on the one that is less concentrated. This pressure compresses the less concentrated fluid and forces it to move. The permeable membrane that separates it from the denser fluid pushes it toward that denser fluid and reduces its concentration. Leaving the less dense environment, the water becomes more concentrated, while also reducing the concentration of the denser environment. A balance between the two fluids is achieved.

The transfer of liquid from one side to the other of the membrane is all the more pronounced the stronger the osmotic pressure, which is to say when there is a greater difference in the concentration of one fluid in comparison with the other. This is how it is that the more concentrated the environment, the more attraction it exerts on the fluid on the other side of the membrane. Conversely, if there is a balance of pressure on either side of a membrane, no exchange will take place.

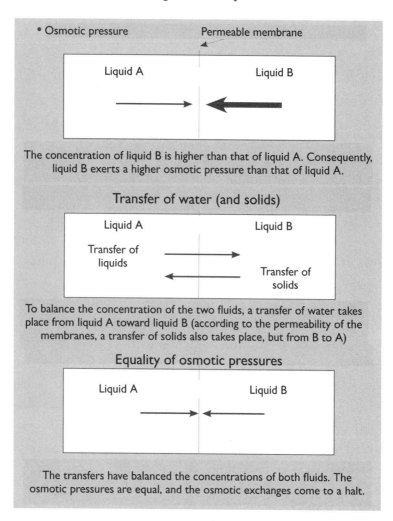

• Osmotic pressure   Permeable membrane

Liquid A   Liquid B

The concentration of liquid B is higher than that of liquid A. Consequently, liquid B exerts a higher osmotic pressure than that of liquid A.

Transfer of water (and solids)

Liquid A   Liquid B

Transfer of
liquids
                                              Transfer of
                                              solids

To balance the concentration of the two fluids, a transfer of water takes place from liquid A toward liquid B (according to the permeability of the membranes, a transfer of solids also takes place, but from B to A)

Equality of osmotic pressures

Liquid A   Liquid B

The transfers have balanced the concentrations of both fluids. The osmotic pressures are equal, and the osmotic exchanges come to a halt.

Osmotic Exchanges

To make its way into the tissues, the water located in the digestive tract must first cross through the walls of the intestines through osmotic transfer in order to enter the bloodstream.

The mucous membrane of the small intestine is carpeted with blood capillaries. The membrane that separates the interior of the intestine from the capillary blood is extremely weak, consisting of only one layer of cells, a layer whose thickness does not exceed 30 thousandths of a millimeter. Osmotic exchanges can therefore take place easily here. This is especially true on this level because the alimentary bolus and the water from beverages remains in contact with the intestinal mucous membrane for a long time.

When a liquid is consumed on its own—that is, when a person drinks without eating—the water taken in by the small intestine is less concentrated than the blood. Blood contains the numerous substances that it transports, such as glucose and minerals, as well as its own constituent elements (red corpuscles and platelets). These solid substances contained in the bloodstream represent up to 10 percent of its weight, compared with one per thousand in water. Osmotic pressure is therefore stronger on the blood side, creating a transfer of water from the intestine into the bloodstream.

The situation does not fundamentally change when drinks are consumed during a meal. The blend of solid foods and liquids obviously produces a fluid whose density is greater than that of water. This density is not very high, though, as alimentary bolus must be fluid enough to advance toward the bottom of the digestive tract. The osmotic pressure exerted by the blood will remain higher, and the passage of water from the intestine into the bloodstream will be achieved easily.

To reverse the osmotic flow—to encourage water to leave the bloodstream and tissues and enter the colon—it is necessary to make the colon's contents more dense. When that is achieved the osmotic pressure exerted by the colon will be stronger than that exerted by the bloodstream. Water will therefore cross through the membranes of the capillaries and enter the colon.

The densification of the liquid content of the colon can be achieved by substances that are hard to assimilate, if they can be assimilated at all. The most common substances capable of moving water from the blood and tissues into the colon are sorbitol and lactose. By remaining in the colon, these substances contribute to increasing the density of the fecal bolus and, thus, the osmotic pressure it exerts. However, if too many of these substances are present they will have too strong an effect. The colon will take in too much water from the blood and surrounding tissues; the stools will liquefy and leave the body in the form of diarrhea. The amount of sorbitol and lactose taken into the body is therefore quite important, and the ideal amount varies greatly from person to person. Each person must find the dosage that works for him- or herself to obtain enough hydration of the stools so they can be easily evacuated, but no more.

Here we will take a more in-depth look at these substances.

HYDROPHILIC SUBSTANCES

Name	Source
Sorbitol	Pears, prunes, peaches, apricots, apples
Lactose	Whey

Sorbitol

Sorbitol, a sugar of plant origin, comes from the *Sorbus aucuparia* (rowan or mountain ash), a tree whose orange berries are rich in the natural sweetener. Sorbitol gives a sweet flavor to foods but is not fattening and does not cause problems for diabetics. It is used to sweeten jams and candies. The recommendation found on packages of cough drops that contain sorbitol is worth noting—it warns consumers from taking too many, as they will have a laxative effect and cause diarrhea by liquefying the stools.

It is this effect that we wish to examine here, to adapt sorbitol to our needs with an adequate dosage.

Source

Sorbitol is primarily found in fruits. Its principal sources are prunes, pears, peaches, apricots, and apples. As shown by the following table, the sorbitol content in these fruits is higher when they are dried, because by drying them the water content is reduced and the concentration of the constituent elements is increased.

SORBITOL CONTENT OF VARIOUS FRUITS
(per 100 grams)

Dried Fruits	Fresh Fruits and Juices
Dried pears (10 g)	Fresh pears, pear juice (2 g)
Dried prunes (8 g)	Fresh plums, prune juice (2 g)
Dried peaches (5 g)	Fresh peaches (1 g)
Dried apricots (5 g)	Fresh apricots (1 g)
Dried apples (3 g)	Fresh apples (0.5 g)
Dates (2 g)	
Dried fruits (blend) (2 g)	

Dried prunes are the fruits that are most often used from this list, even though their sorbitol content is not the highest. The reason for this is that it is not only the presence of sorbitol that gives them their laxative properties; prunes also have a high fiber content. These fibers are soluble. They become charged with large quantities of water, which gives volume to the stools while hydrating them well. It is the combination of these two factors that make prunes so effective and so commonly used. They act on two fundamental causes of constipation: the lack of water and the lack of fiber.

Using Sorbitol to Cure Constipation

Choose one of the fruits from the table above. Given the fact that you should eat it every day, start with a fruit you like and in a form that works for you: dry, fresh, or juiced. Most often these fruits are used in their dried form because they are not available fresh all year long. The effect of this regimen should begin to become noticeable in two or three days. To maintain the effect, continue to eat the selected fruit daily.

Dried fruits are eaten as is or they can be steeped for several hours or overnight. They can be eaten the next day with the juice.

Good to Know

Steeped prunes and figs are more effective than eating these fruits dry.

The time of day is not really important. The chosen fruit can be eaten at breakfast, as a snack, or in the evening. The main

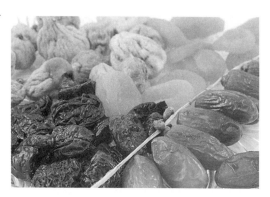

Dates, prunes, and apricots are a few of the fruits that contain sorbitol.

thing is to eat the fruit every day. Incorporating the selected fruit into a specific meal daily is a good way to remember to eat it. Some people eat prunes for breakfast every day; others eat a pear before going to bed.

If you start to tire of eating the selected fruit, opt for another, and continue with that one. People who love variety can change the type of fruit every day. But as these fruits do not all contain the same level of sorbitol, the dosage will need to be changed depending on the fruit.

Dosage

Dosage is important. It is important that you eat enough of the fruit for it to have an effect on stool formation. The dosage is eminently personal, because each person will have a different reaction. Begin with a small dose and gradually increase it every day, until the effects can be seen in the elimination of stools.

For example, start with two prunes for two or three days; then increase the dose to three prunes. After a few weeks the dosage may have to be adjusted upward or downward based on the fruit's effects. If the effects seem to be weakening, the dose will need to be increased; if they are intensifying, lessen the amount of fruit you are eating.

Lactose

As indicated by its name, lactose is a sugar that comes from milk. It is also known as milk sugar. It is actually a double sugar that consists of galactose and glucose.

Lactose has hygroscopic properties, which means it attracts and retains water. During the digestive process, the lactose contained in the dairy products we eat is not entirely digested at the top of the digestive tract. It remains in the form of lactose until it reaches the bottom of the small intestine and the colon. When a substantial amount of lactose has been consumed, it has the potential to help draw water to and retain it in the colon. The hydration this creates thereby facilitates the softening and elimination of stools.

Lactose is digested by a special enzyme. This enzyme is present in a great number of people during childhood but becomes more rare in adults. This is one of the reasons adults have trouble digesting milk, and why a portion of the lactose ingested finds its way to the colon without being transformed. In extreme cases, all the lactose makes its way into the colon. There it liquefies the stools and causes the diarrhea that afflicts individuals who are allergic to lactose. (Obviously the whey regimen discussed below is contraindicated for lactose-intolerant people.)

Practice of the Whey Cure

Whey is a liquid obtained from the manufacture of cheese. The pressured milk that curdles separates into a hard part, known as casein (or fromage blanc), and a liquid part, the whey. This process is easy to observe with fromage blanc in a cheese strainer, where you see both a solid part and a liquid part. This latter is whey. It is slightly transparent and has a yellowish-green color and a sour taste.

Whey must be drunk very fresh, as it alters rapidly at contact with air. It is, however, more difficult to find it in this form. This is the reason the whey regimen is most often practiced with powdered or granular whey (for more see my book *The Whey Prescription*). These forms of whey are produced using modern procedures that preserve its healthful properties. The lactose content in whey can be as high as 75 percent. By mixing the powder with cold or lukewarm water, you get a drinkable form of whey.

Different brands are available. Some offer natural whey, while others have fruit flavors. One company even sells flavored whey candies.

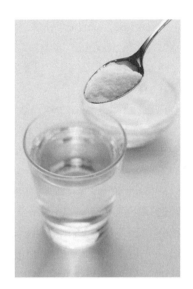

Whey can be reconstituted from dry whey granules.

Dosage

Reconstituted whey is prepared by adding 1 heaping tablespoon of powder to 1 to 2 deciliters of water. It must be drunk immediately after preparing, when it is still quite fresh. If whey is ingested daily, the effects will begin to make themselves felt in two to three days. If this is not the case, the dosage should be increased to meet the body's needs.

You should drink two, three, or four glasses of whey a day, before meals or between them as snacks. Once you determine the number of glasses per day necessary to produce soft stools that are easy to evacuate, that dosage should be maintained.

Observations and Precautions

Some people can experience bloating at the beginning of this therapeutic regimen. When this happens, the regimen should be interrupted for several days and then started again with smaller doses (½ tablespoon of whey, for example), which can be gradually increased.

As noted earlier, this regimen is contraindicated for people who are lactose intolerant.

Other Properties

The beneficial effects of whey are only partially due to its lactose content. The other effect comes from the action of the lactic acid, which has a stimulating effect on peristalsis.

Using Milk Sugar to Cure Constipation

The milk sugar on sale in health stores is composed of 100 percent lactose. It has been extracted from milk and transformed into a powder. Mixed with milk, it produces a slightly sweet beverage with a pleasant flavor.

Dosage

The basic beverage is obtained by mixing 1 tablespoon of lactose with 2 to 3 deciliters of cold or warm water. If drinking this blend once a day is insufficient for obtaining any effect on the consistency of the stools, it should be drunk 2 to 3 times a day. Another means of increasing the dose is to go from 1 level tablespoon to 1 semi-heaping tablespoon, or even a heaping tablespoon. Through trial and error you will eventually discover the necessary dosage for obtaining soft stools that are not at all difficult to eliminate.

Observations and Precautions

Bloating can occur at the beginning of this therapeutic regimen. If this happens, it is a good idea to halt the regimen for several days. When you begin again, start with smaller doses (1 teaspoon rather than 1 tablespoon of powder) that will be increased very gradually.

This regimen is contraindicated for people who are allergic to lactose.

5 The Liver and Constipation

The liver, an organ that is independent of the intestines, plays a fundamental role in the function of the intestines through the secretions it pours into them. In fact, the bile that the liver produces is not simply a digestive juice. Bile also has a decisive effect on intestinal transit, which it stimulates in a variety of ways.

This means that a sluggish liver—a liver that is not producing enough bile to ensure the normal progression of stools through the intestines—can also be a cause of constipation.

THE ROLE OF THE LIVER

Among its many functions, the liver performs the role of purifying the blood of the wastes it carries. It then secretes those wastes in a viscous fluid called bile. Bile is known primarily for its action in the digestion of fats. The bile is transported into the intestines by the bile duct; some bile is forced into the gallbladder, where the bile is stored in reserve to be released for digesting the larger amounts of fats that can occur during a meal. When ingested fats reach this level and require bile from the gallbladder,

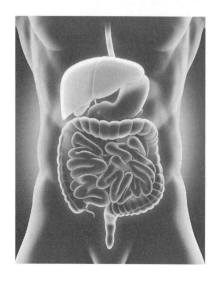

The liver has an important role to play in healthy elimination.

the gallbladder contracts several times to project the bile into the intestines.

Bile emulsifies fats, reducing fats into very tiny droplets that will be broken down by the enzymes of the pancreatic juices. Bile also stimulates intestinal peristalsis. Its action on this level is two-fold: stimulating peristalsis and lubricating the intestines.

Stimulation of Intestinal Peristalsis

As we have seen already, intestinal peristalsis is triggered when the intestines are filled with matter and their walls are distended. But the intestines can also be stimulated to contract by the presence of bile, and this can occur without any intestinal distension.

By its composition, bile has the ability to stimulate the sensitive nerves that are located in the intestinal walls. These nerves then send the signal to the peristaltic muscles to get to work. Bile's presence alone in the intestines therefore has the effect of activating intestinal contractions and encouraging the progression of matter through the digestive tract. In other words, when there is no bile present, no signal will be given. In this case the intestinal peristalsis that is so necessary for digestive and eliminatory processes would only be triggered by the presence of a large amount of roughage, which will stretch the intestinal walls.

The stimulation of the intestines depends on the quantity of bile present. Normally there is always enough. But many people have lazy livers. They suffer from hepatic insufficiency, which is the term used to describe the situation when the liver does not release as much bile as it should. This deficit can vary in scope depending on the individual. The consequence of not enough bile is that the intestine is barely stimulated to work, if at all. The matter that is present in the intestines will only advance through them slowly and with difficulty, drying out and hardening along the way.

Lubrication of the Intestinal Mucous Membranes

Another property of bile is its ability to lubricate the intestines.

The intestines are so often compared to a long tube that it is easy to imagine that their interior walls are smooth, like the texture of a pipe. But this is not the case at all—their inner surfaces are not flat and smooth. The mucous membranes of the small intestine are formed from numerous creases in the intestinal wall called the intestinal villi. These creases give a wrinkled and uneven aspect to the walls, which hinders the free progression of food matter in the intestines.

There are no villi in the colon, but its walls are not smooth, either. They are made uneven by the projections, dents, and furrows created by the muscles contained in its walls. Another cause for their irregular surface is the presence of small glands that protrude from the colon's surface.

A certain braking action therefore hinders the passage of matter in the intestines. To counter this effect, nature provides a lubricant that consists partially of the bile secreted by the liver, which reduces friction and makes the intestinal tract slippery. The lubricant also includes mucus secretions generated by the intestinal walls themselves.

Bile possesses a greasy quality that acts inside the intestines much the same way that oil works to lubricate an engine. Just as a motor can only function correctly when it has enough oil, and that oil is of good quality, the intestines can only advance the matter they contain when there is a sufficient amount of bile present, which must also be of good quality.

The quantity of bile released by a healthy liver on a daily basis can be as high as 1 liter. It moves along with the foods present in the intestines. It forms a deposit on the intestinal walls and lubricates them by its greasy and oily nature. In this way it greatly facilitates the progression of the matter that is pushed forward by the contraction of the peristaltic muscles. Therefore it can be said that there is an efficacious collaboration between bile and peristalsis to ensure a good transit of the matter in the intestines.

For a person with a lazy liver, the quantity of bile produced is not sufficient for lubricating the intestines. The stools advance slowly and with much difficulty, because the peristaltic muscles cannot push the matter forward by themselves. When the stools remain stagnant for too long, they harden and become sticky, and thereby cause constipation.

Another important factor to consider is the quality of the bile. People who have a high level of toxins in their bodies from overeating, smoking, drinking alcohol, taking medications, and so forth will have bile that contains more toxins than normal. These toxins make the bile both thicker and denser; it loses its oily character and can no longer lubricate the intestinal mucous membranes as well. The situation can be compared to the proper functioning of an engine—once the oil has collected too much waste from the friction caused by the motor's parts rubbing against one another, it becomes overloaded and can no longer perform its job properly. The purpose for the periodic emptying of oil from the motor is to replace the thick oil with oil that is pure and slippery.

When it comes to the liver, this "emptying" process amounts to detoxifying the liver so that the bile can recover its normal fluidity. This can be done in a variety of ways that we shall take a look at later.

The congestion of the liver that leads to constipation is often caused by constipation itself. In fact, the nutritive substances that foods release during the digestive process enter the blood capillaries located in the intestinal walls. These capillaries join together to form the portal vein, which transports its contents into the liver. This is how everything that is absorbed by the intestines first passes through the liver before making its way into the rest of the body.

Normally, these nutrients are characteristically small molecules. Sometimes, though, the substances extracted from the food we ingest are toxins, which are larger molecules. When the intestinal mucous membranes that act as the filter are damaged, the mucous membranes will let not only the substances that are useful to the body into the blood; they will also let in wastes and poisons that would normally not be able to enter because of their size.

The mesh of the mucous membrane filter is damaged by prolonged contact of toxins with the intestinal mucous membranes, and by the irritating and aggressive poisons created by matter fermenting and putrefying inside the intestines. These fermentations and putrefactions are the results of an overly slow intestinal transit, which is to say they are the consequences of constipation.

THE SYMPTOMS OF LIVER SLUGGISHNESS (HEPATIC INSUFFICIENCY)

To determine if liver sluggishness is one of the causes of your constipation, it is necessary to recognize the signs that reveal when the liver is not working well. They are quite easy to observe. It should be noted that a person suffering from a hepatic weakness will present one, but more often several, of the following symptoms:

- difficulty digesting fats: fried foods, eggs, cream, and so forth
- digestive troubles in general
- nausea
- swelling and heaviness around the belly
- gas, bloating
- furred mouth, coated tongue
- bad breath
- loss of appetite
- fatigue, lack of enthusiasm
- stools shaped like goat droppings
- stools too light in color due to the absence of bilirubin
- stools that float in the toilet because of an insufficient digestion of fats

PRACTICAL SOLUTIONS

LIVER STIMULATION

When constipation is due to reduced liver function, the treatment plan to follow should not target the intestines; it should be focused on the liver. It is the liver that is responsible for the slowdown in the intestinal transit because of its weak production of bile.

The most effective means for stimulating the liver in
its work are the use of medicinal plants
and a hot-water bottle.

MEDICINAL PLANTS

Medicinal plants for the liver are known as "hepatic plants," or plants "that drain the liver and gallbladder." They act by stimulating the liver to filter more wastes out of the blood, which will increase the quantity of bile produced. In the best-case scenario, bile production will double. This means that the intestines will receive much more bile for lubricating their walls and for stimulating intestinal peristalsis. Furthermore, hepatic plants increase the gallbladder's ability to contract and thereby eject the bile it has temporarily stored. The result is an increased amount of bile in the intestines.

The congestion of the liver by wastes and poisons, which has led to hepatic insufficiency, is a process that occurs over time. Years of gradual intoxication obviously cannot be turned around by a therapeutic regimen lasting several days. Practice shows that it is necessary to take hepatic plants for a period of one to three months, three times a day, before meals. With these regular doses repeated over time, the liver will gradually get rid of the wastes that are burdening it and become less and less congested. It will regain its strength and recover its normal function.

Here are three plants that are especially effective for stimulating the liver to perform its work. The dosage indicated must be adapted to fit your personal needs. Start with small doses and increase them gradually. When intestinal transit has been restored, maintain this dosage for one to three months.

Artichoke (Cynara scolymus)

The part that is used in therapy is not the heart of the flower, which is customarily eaten, but the leaves.

Infusion

10 grams of artichoke leaves per 1 liter of water; steep for 10 minutes. This makes a very bitter tea. Drink three cups a day.

Gel Caps

1 or 2 gel caps, 3 times a day.

Mother Tincture

30 to 50 drops, 3 times a day.

Black Radish (Raphanus sativus)

The flesh of this radish is white; its skin is black. It is an excellent stimulant for the liver and gallbladder. Its use in cooking is highly recommended.

Vial of Black Radish Juice

1 or 2 (10–15 ml) vials a day.

Gel Caps

1 or 2 gel caps, 3 times a day.

Mother Tincture

30 to 40 drops, 3 times a day.

Rosemary (Rosmarinus officinalis)

A bush native to the Mediterranean, rosemary is covered with little leaves that highly stimulate the liver. They can double bile production. Its use in cooking is highly recommended.

Infusion

1 teaspoon of leaves per 1 cup, steep for 15 minutes. Drink two to three cups a day.

Gel Caps

1 or 2 gel caps, 3 times a day.

Mother Tincture

20 to 40 drops, 3 times a day.

THE HOT-WATER BOTTLE

A loss of heat in the area of the hepatic gland due to fatigue and weakened conditions will reduce the liver's ability to work. It so happens that cold has a vasoconstrictive effect on the blood capillaries. They shrink in diameter, which slows down blood circulation in the liver. This hampers bile production.

To fight against hepatic insufficiency, nothing works as well as placing a hot-water bottle over the liver. This will allow the organ to get the heat it needs to work actively. The hot-water bottle is a rubber cushion equipped with an opening that can be hermetically sealed with a cork. Fill the bottle with hot water from the tap and place it over the area of the liver. It will transmit its heat to the organ. The liver's temperature will rise, and its functioning, which had been slowed, will resume its normal rhythm, and in some cases even intensify.

Instructions
- Place the bottle filled with hot water over the liver.
- Keep it there for 15 to 30 minutes.
- Do this one to three times a day, preferably after meals.
- This regimen should be followed for at least one month.

6 Constipating Foods and Medications

Some constipation is due to the consumption of food or ingestion of medications that have constipating effects. Depending on the case, they will create constipation in an individual who was previously not suffering from it, or they will make an existing case of constipation worse.

The constipating effects of certain foods and medications are exhibited by a decelerating effect on:

- the secretions of mucus by the intestinal walls
- intestinal peristalsis

In the first case, the responsible agents are foods and various medicinal plants that have an astringent effect. In the second case, medications are the primary culprit, as they inhibit the parasympathetic nervous system, which is responsible for triggering peristalsis.

We will examine both these points in detail to explain the mechanisms that are brought into play, and to present the foods and medications that trigger them.

However, it is necessary to make an important observation here. When someone who has not been suffering from constipation becomes constipated after beginning to eat food or take medications that can cause constipation, the elimination of those substances will be enough for the person's intestines to begin functioning normally again. On the other hand, when someone is already constipated and their problems increase by the ingestion of food or medications, treatment should focus on eliminating the food substances or medication as well as dealing with the root cause of the constipation.

DECELERATING EFFECT ON MUCUS SECRETIONS

The walls of the small intestine and colon are carpeted with glands that secrete a free-flowing fluid. This liquid contains digestive juices as well as a mucus that acts as a lubricant.

A lubricant is a greasy substance. It reduces friction by creating a smooth surface for two elements to rub against one another. We use a lubricant in a motor so that its various parts can move easily; we also use a lubricant to loosen stuck or blocked screws and bolts. In the intestines, the secreted mucus serves the stools as a lubricant so that the stools do not become stuck to the intestinal walls but instead glide by them easily. It also plays a protective role. The greasy coating it forms over the intestinal mucous membranes protects them from more or less dry or aggressive matter that is present in the intestines.

The intestines produce 3 liters of mucus-containing secretions a day. This is a fairly large quantity, especially when compared to the volume of other secretions of the digestive tract (1.5 liters of digestive juices, 1 liter of saliva, 1 liter of bile). These various secretions are not evacuated with the stools but are, for the most part, reabsorbed by the body and reutilized.

The pace of secretion of mucus by the intestinal walls can be slowed, however, by certain substances present in food or medicinal plants. These substances, known as astringents, cause the mesh-like lining of the mucous membranes to tighten, especially those of the intestines. Instead of the cellular juxtaposition that keeps each cell a short distance from each neighboring cell in the mucous membrane, the cells become tightly bunched next to each other. This hinders and even blocks the passageway through which the glands spill their secretions. When these secretions happen less frequently, the lubricating effect is reduced, which consequently slows down the intestinal transit.

A well-known example of an astringent substance is the tannin used to treat leather. By "retightening" the surface of the leather, it becomes rot resistant and can be kept for a very long time. This phenomenon of leather retightening is similar to what takes place on the surface of the skin when we get goose bumps.

The action of astringents tightens the mesh-like lining of the intestines and slow secretions from the intestinal walls.

The skin contracts and thereby reduces the exchanges between the inside and outside of the body.

Foods Rich in Astringent Substances

Various foods have a high content of astringent substances, and therefore also have a constipating effect. This effect can manifest in a more or less pronounced way, depending on the person. Generally speaking, it is necessary to eat these foods on a regular basis for a slowdown of the intestinal transit to take place, but sometimes eating one of these foods once is all it takes. However, in this latter case the constipation will only be temporary.

Foods with constipating effects are:

- bananas
- barbary figs (the seeds)
- blueberries
- fresh apricots
- lemon or lemon juice in excess quantities (for some people)
- loquats
- pomegranates
- quinces
- red wine
- white rice (for some people)
- wild blackberries

Good to Know

Astringent foods are not essential for life. To treat the constipation that their consumption has caused, it is enough to remove the foods from your diet and replace them with other foods.

Medicinal Plants with Constipating Effects

Various medicinal plants have an astringent effect that has been used advantageously to tighten the tissue of an organ, like those of a blood vessel in the case of varicose veins or bleeding. A person who takes a remedy such as an herbal tea, gel caps, or a tincture based on these plants several times a day and continues taking them for several weeks or months will see as an unwanted side effect a significant slowdown of his or her intestinal transit. In fact, astringent substances not only go to the ailing part of the body—the varicose vein, for example—but scatter throughout the entire body. Consequently, they will also make their way into the intestines.

A person who becomes constipated shortly after beginning to take medicinal plants should check to see whether they have astringent properties or not. The most common astringent plants are:

- agrimony
- beech
- blueberry
- celandine
- comfrey
- dead nettle
- goldenrod
- herb Robert
- Indian chestnut
- lady's mantle
- loosestrife
- milfoil
- nettle
- oak
- poplar
- shepherd's purse
- tormentil
- walnut
- willow
- yarrow

Advice

To prevent needing to interrupt a treatment using one or more medicinal plants, you should try to find other plants with the same therapeutic effects that do not have the constipating side effects. If you are unable to find them, you can address the constipating effect by taking plant laxatives (see chapter 11).

OTHER FACTORS THAT INHIBIT SECRETION

Alcohol Abuse

Alcoholic beverages have a paralyzing effect on the mucous membranes of the intestines—in fact, alcohol dries out and attacks these mucous membranes. Those who drink alcoholic beverages on a regular basis can suffer from chronic inflammation. It so happens that over the long term this inflammation will lead to the deterioration of the tissues involved. To protect themselves from the assault of alcohol, they will harden, which gradually creates sclerosis. The intestinal mucous membranes will be "sealed" this way, in the same way they are by the action of astringent substances. Mucus secretions will be poor, and the intestinal transit will be greatly slowed down.

When the alcoholic beverage in question is red wine, it will add the astringent effect of the tannins the red wine contains.

Clay Taken Internally

Clay is a remedy that is used commonly in natural medicine. It has beneficial effects for most people, but it can sometimes have a constipating effect when taken orally.

Powdered clay is swallowed with water to treat gastritis, stomach ulcers, and enteritis but is also used to detoxify the body in general. Clay possesses strong absorbent properties, which means it easily attracts substances that are around it and fixes them to itself. This property is beneficial for neutralizing gastric juices, toxins, or poisons. But it is not so beneficial when it has this same effect on the intestines' mucus secretions.

Clay will, in fact, neutralize secretions too heavily in some people's bodies. The lubricating properties of mucus will no longer manifest, and the intestinal transit will slow down. Another drawback of clay's neutralizing ability is that it can suck up too much of the water present in the colon. This will cause the fecal bolus to dry out. The stools will become hard and difficult to eliminate.

Good to Know

The constipating effect of clay can sometimes be compensated for by drinking a lot of water during the therapeutic regimen. If this has no effect, you should halt the clay regimen.

HINDERING EFFECTS OF MEDICATIONS ON INTESTINAL PERISTALSIS

Certain medications hinder intestinal peristalsis by targeting the aspects of the nervous system responsible for peristalsis.

The functioning of the intestines is under the jurisdiction of the autonomic nervous system. This system consists of two branches:

- the sympathetic system—this aspect of the nervous system reduces secretions, slows peristalsis, and reduces the opening of the sphincters
- the parasympathetic system—this aspect of the nervous system increases secretions, stimulates peristalsis, and encourages the sphincters to open

These two systems are antagonistic—when one is activated the other is quiet. Thanks to this predominance of activity of one system over another, the intestines will be stimulated in certain functions (digestion, for example) and restrained in others (such

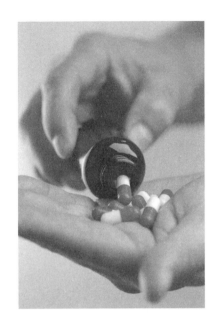

Certain medications can hinder intestinal peristalsis.

as in elimination), or vice versa, depending on the body's needs at a given moment.

Some medications will have a sharply inhibiting factor on the parasympathetic nervous system. The technical way to say this is that they have an anticholinergic effect, because they block the release of acetylcholine by the nerve fibers of the parasympathetic system. This substance is a chemical mediator—an intermediary for the transmission of nerve impulses toward the receptor organs, in this case the intestines. The nerve impulse sent to the intestines by the parasympathetic nervous system only reaches these organs thanks to acetylcholine. If this substance is absent, the order that has been given by the nervous system will not be carried out.

When medications with an anticholinergic action are taken, they bring about a sharp reduction in the pace of intestinal peristalsis. The blocking effect of these medications will consequently cause:

- a reduction in the mucus secretion by the intestinal walls, which will deprive the stools of the lubricating effect that helps them advance through the intestines
- reduced intestinal peristalsis, which will hinder the advance of fecal matter
- an increase in the tone of the sphincters, like those of the anus, which will make the elimination of stools more difficult

Medications That Encourage Constipation
Among these medications, we find:

- antipsychotics (also known as neuroleptics) with an anticholinergic effect
- sleeping pills
- antidepressants
- anticonvulsant anxiolytics (antianxiety drugs)
- opioid analgesics (painkillers)
- antiparkinson drugs
- antispasmodics
- anticholinergic bronchodilators
- anticholinergic antihistamines
- antidiarrheal drugs

Advice

As treatments based on these kinds of medication generally should not be interrupted, it is necessary to take a laxative to compensate for their constipating effects (see chapter 11).

OTHER FACTORS THAT HINDER PERISTALSIS

Laxatives

Paradoxically, laxatives are among the medications that can encourage constipation, but only when they are taken in excess. Their effect is to vigorously stimulate intestinal peristalsis. When this stimulation is only occasional or temporary, the peristaltic muscles can recover after their exertion. But when used too frequently—if not to say regularly—the peristaltic muscles no longer enjoy the recovery time they need. They become exhausted. They will gradually weaken and finally reach the point where they are no longer able to perform their job properly. Intestinal transit will lag, and constipation will become solidly established.

> The overuse of laxatives exhausts the intestines and leads to constipation.

Advice

1. One solution consists of replacing laxatives with enemas, as their action is less tiring on the intestines.
2. Another possibility is to use gentle and nonirritating laxatives, such as whey or prunes.
3. But the true solution consists of acting on the primary and profound causes of constipation: the lack of roughage, the lack of liquid, the lack of bile, and so forth.

7 The Abdominal Muscles and Constipation

The muscles play a very important role in the proper functioning of the intestines. They are active not only in the process of intestinal peristalsis, but also in the process of evacuation (defecation).

The peristaltic muscles push the matter in the intestines forward, in order to help this matter reach its terminal point, the anus. However, this push is not sufficient on its own to ensure the evacuation of the stools out of the body. The anus, in fact, constitutes a narrow passage that cannot be traversed so easily. An additional pressure to enable the stools to be expelled from the body is necessary—this pressure is provided by the abdominal muscles. When they are in good tone, intestinal elimination is achieved easily. But when they are weak and lacking vigor, defecation is performed poorly. In our modern day, which is characterized by a sedentary lifestyle, this is quite common; hence the large number of people who suffer from constipation. In these cases, the solution consists of reinvigorating the muscles involved.

When the peristaltic and abdominal muscles are well toned, intestinal elimination is performed easily.

But before explaining how to proceed in practice, let's take a look at the different muscles that come into play here.

THE PERISTALTIC MUSCLES

The peristaltic muscles were first introduced in chapter 3. They consist of two different kinds of muscle, both of which are located in the intestinal walls. The bulk of the longitudinal muscles are found on the surface of the intestinal walls. They run lengthwise, their fibers oriented in the direction of the intestines. Their fibers are oriented in such a way that when they contract, the matter present in the intestines is pushed forward, toward the exit.

The second type of muscles are the circular or annular muscles that are in the deeper layers of the intestinal walls. As their name indicates, these muscles are ring-like in shape; they are arranged throughout the entire length of the intestines. Their fibers are perpendicular to the direction that the food matter follows. By contracting, they reduce the diameter of the intestinal tract and even close it.

By contracting one after the other, these muscle rings compel the matter present in the intestines to head toward the end of the intestines. But the circular muscles do not only act in this manner. The succession of contractions can work in the opposite direction; these are called antiperistaltic contractions. They push the food matter backward for a short distance. This makes it possible to retain foods for a longer period in one part of the intestines to ensure that they are perfectly digested before the food moves further down the intestinal tract.

The two movements I just described can also combine in a

segment of the intestines. The foods are not pushed along but remain in one spot and are mixed together by the kneading action of the intestinal muscles. The purpose of these segmentation contractions is to break down the food into tinier pieces, with an eye to facilitating their digestion.

The longitudinal and annular peristaltic muscles are smooth muscles. Contrary to striated muscles, which we will discuss later, the smooth muscles are not under the control of our conscious will. We are not able to *make* them move like we can our striated muscles, such as our biceps. The characteristic feature of the smooth muscles is to perform slow, powerful contractions. In fact, the progression of foods through the intestines must be slow so that the digestive process has the time it needs to do its work properly.

THE DEFECATING OR ABDOMINAL MUSCLES

Thanks to intestinal peristalsis, matter advances into the small intestine, then into the ascending colon, transverse colon, and, finally, to the descending colon. This latter part of the colon is composed of different parts that I will briefly describe to facilitate understanding the process of evacuation.

The descending colon, which is located on the left side of the abdomen, first descends vertically, then makes two turns, which gives it the shape of an S, hence its name at this juncture—the sigmoid colon. The sigmoid colon is followed by the rectum, a bulge in the intestinal tract that makes it possible for a certain amount of matter to collect. It is also called the rectal ampulla (or ampulla recti). This ampulla terminates in the anus.

Through the action of the peristaltic muscles of the descending colon, the fecal matter is pushed into the sigmoid colon, which straightens out as it fills with matter, losing its S shape. The peristaltic contractions continue and cause the fecal matter to

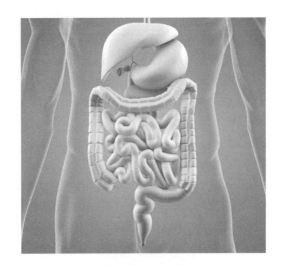

The rectum is a bulge in the lower intestinal tract where digested food matter collects.

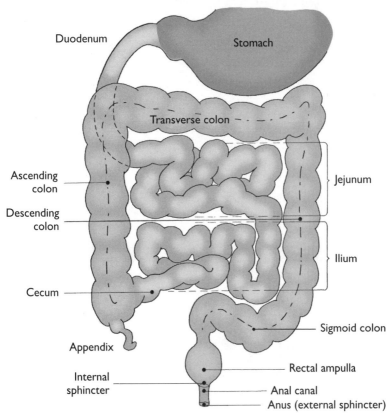

Duodenum

Stomach

Transverse colon

Ascending colon

Jejunum

Descending colon

Ilium

Cecum

Sigmoid colon

Appendix

Rectal ampulla

Internal sphincter

Anal canal

Anus (external sphincter)

A schematic of the digestive system

descend into the rectal ampulla. The walls of the rectum become distended by the arrival of the stools, which trigger the sensation of needing to defecate. The last passage through which the stools need to move in order to exit the body is the anus. This latter is a sphincter, which is to say an annular muscle. When contracted, it keeps the anus closed.

Contrary to the other muscles of the intestines, those of the anus are striated and are consequently subject to our will. If conditions are not favorable, we can decide to counter our need to defecate by intentionally holding the anal sphincter closed. When we decide to respond positively to our body's signal, all we need to do is intentionally relax the sphincter. This means that the exit door is open. But in order for the matter that is ready to be eliminated to actually be evacuated, it must be expelled toward the outside. This expulsion takes place thanks to a sustained contraction, not by the peristaltic muscles but by the abdominal muscles. Their role is to compress the lower part of the colon to force the stools to exit, in the same way we squeeze a tube to cause its contents to burst out.

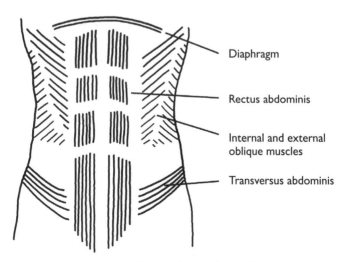

Diaphragm

Rectus abdominis

Internal and external oblique muscles

Transversus abdominis

The abdominal muscles

Four different kinds of abdominal muscles combine their efforts to create this compression.

- **The rectus abdominis muscle:** This vertical muscle begins at the front of the rib cage, in the area of the sternum, and goes down to the pubis. This muscle is quite visible. It has been described as looking like a chocolate bar because its dents are easy to see and resemble those of a chocolate bar.
- **The external and internal obliques:** Lateral and oblique, these muscles run from the rib cage toward the iliac crests (the hip bone).
- **Transversus abdominis muscle:** This is a deep-lying and large muscle that wraps horizontally from the back of the body to the front. It travels through the entire lower abdomen, enveloping it like a large belt. This characteristic has led to its being called the "strap muscle."
- **Diaphragm:** This is a dome-shaped muscle that is located above the abdomen.

These muscles are striated and are therefore subject to our will. They can, however, partially function in an autonomous manner, as in the act of evacuation. Contrary to the smooth muscles, these muscles contract rapidly, which allows the prompt and expeditious process that is the evacuation of stools.

THE EVACUATION OF STOOLS

The final push on the terminating part of the intestines is carried out in the following way. Above them, the diaphragm drops and tightens, thereby exerting pressure downward on the intestinal mass. This pressure is applied by forcing exhalation against the closed glottis. The rectus abdominis muscle also contracts, compressing the intestinal mass backward. The oblique muscles and the transversus also go into action and compress the intestinal mass from the sides. Surrounded on all sides but the bottom, the matter present in the final part of the colon can only move through the sole path that remains open: the anus. The matter then leaves the intestines by virtue of one or two simultaneous pushes by the different muscles involved in the evacuation of stools.

Everything therefore works together to reduce the available space in the abdomen to the maximum extent possible, to compress the abdomen and push the matter out of the body. The abdominal muscles work independently, without willful effort. The abdominal muscles are also the muscles that people suffering from constipation willfully contract for pushing purposes. They also palpate the abdominal muscles, placing their hands on both sides of the lower abdomen for the purpose of reinforcing the pressure exerted by their weakened muscles. Sometimes these efforts lead to success and the colon empties, but not always.

While intentionally contracting these muscles—pushing, in other words—is sometimes a legitimate help, it does carry the threat of doing it too energetically and over too long a period of time. The pressure that is being exerted will then have a negative effect on the blood vessels located in the anus and rectum. Their walls will become stretched out and weakened, resulting in the formation of varicose veins, known as hemorrhoids when they occur in this region of the body.

THE NECESSITY OF GOOD MUSCLE TONE

Numerous smooth and striated muscles enter into play to achieve the elimination of stools. However, this process will not work properly unless these muscles are in a good functional state. This is unfortunately not the state of the abdominal musculature of some people suffering with constipation. Their stools are already difficult to eject because they are hard and dry. But this drawback is accompanied by another problem—the muscles responsible for elimination are too weak. They would already have trouble eliminating normal stools, so hard and dry stools pose an even greater challenge.

Like all the muscles of the body, the abdominal muscles can be in a more or less good state of functioning. A person who regularly places demands on the muscles through physical activity will keep the muscles in good tone and functioning at a high level of performance. The reduced activity of a sedentary lifestyle, on the other hand, will lead to the weakening of a person's muscles. Because no demands are made on the muscles, they lose volume and tone. Because the flow of fluids through the muscles is stagnant, they start collecting deposits of fats and toxins, further hindering their ability to react to solicitation.

This weakening of our muscular system is due to our lifestyle. Technological progress has led to the construction of innumerable machines that work in our stead: cars, elevators, washing machines, vacuum cleaners, and so on. The reduction of manual occupations and the increase of sedentary activities is also a contributing factor. The use of machines to help us perform daily tasks is a good thing, but in my opinion this help has gone too far, resulting in a lack of demand on our muscles that leads to a weakening of the muscle system overall, and that of the peristaltic and abdominal muscles in particular.

This muscular weakness is the actual cause for a high number of the cases of constipation in the current population. It also explains the frequency of colon prolapse now. The colon is held in place by muscles; once these muscles weaken, the colon stops

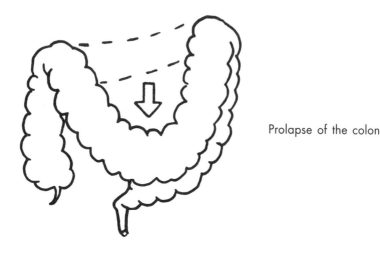

Prolapse of the colon

being maintained in its proper place. This is especially true with the transverse colon. When this section of the abdominal body weakens it causes a prolapse of the colon. The colon curves downward before climbing back up, which cannot help but impede the progression of the stools.

The problem of a lack of tone in the intestinal and abdominal muscles can only be solved by strengthening these muscles, which means using and exercising them again.

SMOOTH MUSCLES, STRIATED MUSCLES

The reeducation of striated muscles is achievable through appropriate exercise, as these muscles are subject to our will. But what can be done for the peristaltic muscles—smooth muscles controlled by the autonomic nervous system, not by our will?

The problem seems insolvable, as even with intense effort we cannot compel these muscles to work. A solution does exist, though. In fact, the peristaltic muscles are stimulated once they begin becoming distended. Their stretching and deformation by the presence of large quantities of roughage have already been mentioned as triggering elements for peristalsis. It so happens that the distension and stimulation of the peristaltic muscles can also be stimulated through abdominal exercise. In fact, by contracting the abdominal muscles (rectus abdominis, internal and external oblique, and transversus abdominis muscles) you pull, compress, and stretch the peristaltic muscles, which gives these muscles the signal to go to work. In other words, the activation through exercise of the abdominal muscles (which are subject to our will) automatically leads to the stimulation of the peristaltic muscles (not subject to our will). The final result is that the peristaltic muscles will become stronger and more responsive.

The effect of the striated muscles on the smooth muscles explains the urge to defecate that happens for some people as soon as they begin to engage in physical activity.

The action exercised by the peristaltic muscles can also be obtained by massage. In fact, by stretching, kneading, and compressing the intestines, massage distends their walls and thereby triggers the activity of the peristaltic muscles. By being made to go to work, and on a regular basis when massages are daily, these muscles will develop and achieve better tone. Over time they will regain their capability to work normally.

There is a third means of stimulating the peristaltic muscles. It works through the nerves and not through the muscles, but as the process is similar, I will touch on it here. It involves massaging the reflex zones of the feet. The reflex zones are small surfaces of our skin that are home to nerve endings connected to specific internal organs. One region of the body that has a wealth of these zones is the soles of the feet. All the organs of the body are represented there, including the intestines. By massaging these zones, the corresponding organ is stimulated and therefore strengthened and toned.

PRACTICAL SOLUTIONS

EXERCISES FOR STRENGTHENING THE ABDOMINAL AND PERISTALTIC MUSCLES

Here I present exercises for the abdominal muscles only, since there are no exercises that affect the peristaltic muscles directly. However, the work performed by the abdominal muscles calls on the peristaltic muscles to work automatically.

To strengthen and develop the abdominal muscles, it is necessary to subject them to repeated contractions. In this way, the pace of blood circulation and cellular exchanges is intensified, causing the muscle fiber to increase in volume and get stronger. The exercises that put demand on the abdominal muscles consequently consist of several series of contractions, each series being punctuated by a period of rest. In the beginning, perform each series only a few times, increasing the number of repetitions as you continue to train. This will make it possible to perform a series of 10, 20, or 40 contractions followed by a brief moment to recuperate. Each series is repeated two or three times before moving on to the next series.

One session will include three exercises. Each exercise acts on a different muscle: one on the rectus abdominis muscle, another on the internal and external oblique muscles, and the last on the transversus abdominis muscle. Practice the first three exercises every day for a period of one to two weeks, then move on to three different exercises. Remember that the exercises you feel are the most tiresome to perform are those that you likely need the most. In fact, the pain you may feel in performing an exercise stems from the fact that the muscles needed to perform that exercise are weak. These are thus the muscles that you need to develop.

The reeducation of the intestinal muscles will take time.

But through regular practice over a period of months you will obtain good abdominal muscle tone. The result will be the restoration of good intestinal function. It would be a good idea to not restrict yourself to only doing abdominal exercises, but also to include aerobic activities—walking, bike riding, or swimming, for example—to combat the overall muscle softening that is engendered by a sedentary lifestyle.

Here are the three major groups of exercises for toning the abdominal muscles. This list is not exhaustive, as there are many good exercise protocols for the abdomen.

Good to Know

I recommend that you continue to do these exercises even after you are no longer suffering from constipation.

Exercises for the Rectus Abdominis Muscle

1. Scissors

Starting position: Sit on the ground, legs stretched long. Recline your upper body backward, and prop yourself up on your forearms.
Movement: Move each leg alternately up and down in a rhythmic motion, keeping both legs straight.

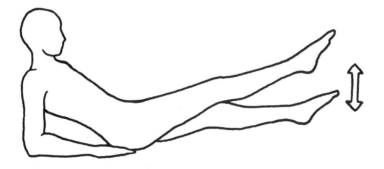

Scissors exercise for the rectus abdominis

2. Bicycle

Starting position: Sit on the ground, legs stretched long. Recline your upper body backward, and prop yourself up on your forearms.
Movement: Make alternating semicircular movements with your legs, as if you were peddling a bike.

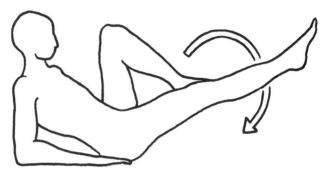

Bicycle exercise for the rectus abdominis

3. The Oars

Starting position: Sit on the ground, legs stretched long. Recline your upper body backward, and prop yourself up on your forearms.
Movement 1 (easy version): Stretch one leg out straight and then bend the other in alternation.
Movement 2 (harder version): Bend both legs at the same time and then stretch them out straight together.

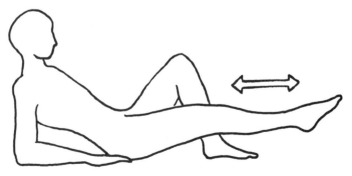

Oars exercise (easy version) for the rectus abdominis

4. Sit-Ups

Starting position: Lie on your back with your calves on a chair. Your calves and thighs should form a right angle. Clasp your hands behind your head.

Movement: Raise your upper body toward your knees. Relax back into the starting position, then repeat.

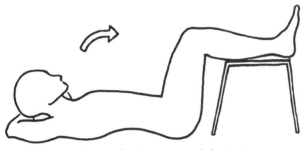

Sit-ups for the rectus abdominis

5. Sit-Ups (harder version)

Starting position: Lie on your back with your knees slightly bent, your feet braced beneath a piece of furniture or a radiator. Clasp your hands behind your head.

Movement: Raise your body from the prone position and bring your forehead over your knees. Relax back into the starting position and then repeat.

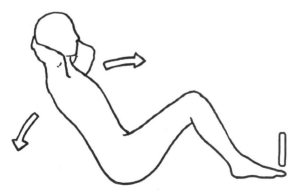

A more demanding version of sit-ups

Exercises for the Internal and External Oblique Muscles

1. Lateral Swing of the Torso

Starting position: Stand erect with both hands clasped behind your head.

Movement 1: Swing your torso in alternation to the left and to the right. Inhale on the right and exhale on the left for a series of movements, and then change the inhale and exhale cycle, inhaling on the left and exhaling on the right.

Movement 2 (harder version): Make the same movements but with your arms stretched above your head, or with a heavy object (a large book, for example) held at the nape of your neck.

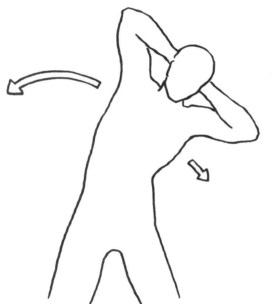

Lateral swings for the internal and external obliques

2. Lateral Swings while Lying Prone

Starting point: Lie on your back with your arms spread out to form a cross. Bend your knees so your thighs are vertical and your calves make a right angle to your thighs.

Movement: Swing your legs in alternation to the left and right.

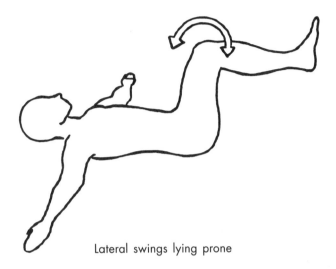

Lateral swings lying prone

3. Cross Swings

Starting point: Lie on your back with your hands clasped behind your head. Your legs should be slightly raised and bent.

Movement: Swing forward to bring your left elbow over your right knee, and then alternate, bringing your right elbow to your left knee.

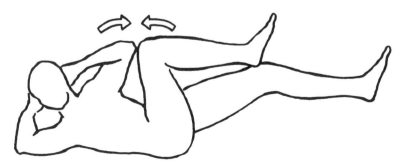

Cross swings for the internal and external obliques

Exercises for the Transversus Abdominis Muscle

1. Retracting the Belly, Prone Position

Starting point: Lie on your back with your hands placed over your torso, your legs bent.

Movement: Pressing your lower back firmly on the ground, exhale and push your navel in toward your spinal column. Maintain for 10 to 20 seconds. Relax, then repeat.

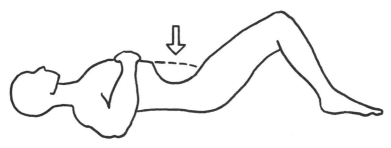

Retracting the belly in prone position, for the transversus abdominis

2. Retracting the Belly, Upright Position

Starting point: Stand with your back against the wall.

Movement 1: Breathe in deeply; then, while holding your breath, push your belly forward for several seconds. Next, exhale slowly (10 seconds) while sucking in your belly, bringing your navel toward your spinal column.

Movement 2: This exercise can also be done while seated.

MASSAGES FOR STRENGTHENING THE PERISTALTIC MUSCLES

Contrary to an organ such as the kidneys, which are protected by the rib cage, the intestines can be touched and palpated through the belly, which is formed of soft tissues. All you need to do is lie down on your back and relax the abdominal muscles in order to massage the peristaltic muscles of the intestines.

The most common massages are self-massages, massages that are easy for anyone to perform effectively on him- or herself. The massage given by a professional massage therapist will of course be much more effective, but as a general rule it is difficult for most people to fit a masseuse visit into their daily schedule, especially for the number of times required for these massages to be effective in remedying constipation.

Intestinal Rub Down

The most often-used massage manipulation is the rub down. This involves applying circular pressure with the fist or fingertips on the region being treated. When this region is the intestines, which measure a number of feet in length, the rub down is performed along the entire length of the intestines. Rub a small portion of the colon for 5 to 10 seconds; then move on to the neighboring section, and so on. Start on the right, in the area where the appendix is located, and gradually move up the length of the ascending

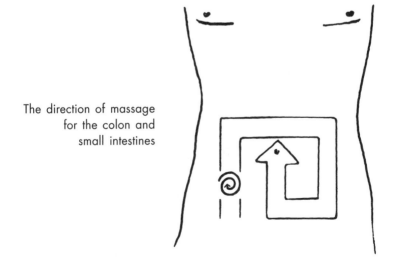

The direction of massage
for the colon and
small intestines

colon. Continue horizontally on the transverse colon toward the left hip; then massage down the descending colon.

Proceed in the same way with the intestines located inside the frame formed by the three parts of the colon. This area can be reached by massaging the zone around the navel.

During a session of self-massage, you will sometimes discover that certain parts of the intestines are hard or tight. Do not hesitate to work more on these zones to soften and relax them. A session of massaging your intestines should take five to ten minutes. It must be done every day. The first effects will manifest after several days, but for more long-lasting effects, you should plan on doing this for several weeks.

Massage with a Tennis Ball

This massage is performed with a tennis ball. Place the ball on the belly. Press the ball into the belly as you move it along the course of the colon for three to five minutes. Move in a clockwise direction, for this is the direction of the colon transit. Daily rep-

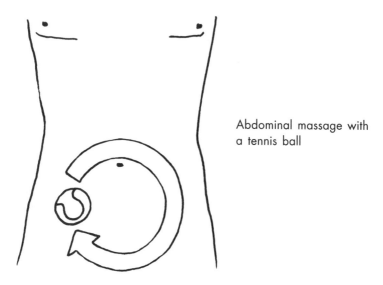

Abdominal massage with a tennis ball

etition of this massage for a period of several weeks will reawaken the slumbering peristalsis of the constipated intestines.

Reflex Zone Massage

Rubbing a specific reflex zone of the feet for a period of several minutes will stimulate its corresponding organ—the intestines in our case—to start working. Blood circulation and cellular exchanges in the peristaltic muscles will be intensified. This will cause them to contract, triggering the peristaltic movements of the intestines.

Through repeated stimulations over the course of a foot massage session and from one session to the next, the peristaltic muscles should be roused from their torpor and become activated. They will gradually get stronger, thanks to the exercise they are receiving. Over time, they will begin to work normally again.

To practice, rub some oil or cream into the reflex zones you plan to treat to facilitate the fingers' ability to glide smoothly on the surface and protect the skin, as it is going to be the subject of repeated friction. This massage is best performed with the thumb.

The following diagram shows where the reflex zones of the colon and small intestine are located on each foot. The entire trajectory of the colon and entire surface of the small intestine zones should be rubbed vigorously on the soles of both feet. Both zones can be massaged at the same time. Some parts will be painful when pressure is applied. These represent irritated areas or areas that are affected by spasms. They should be worked on for a longer period of time but also, in the beginning, with a more delicate touch.

The first sessions should only last a few minutes (two to five minutes); their duration can be gradually increased to ten to twenty minutes. This gradual approach is necessary, as it will allow the intestines to become accustomed little by little to a more intense rate of activity. Beginning with a fifteen-minute session,

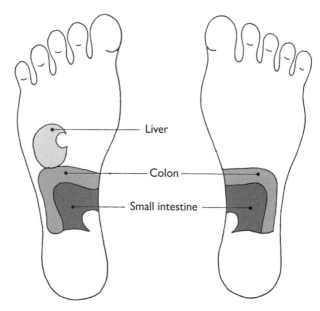

The reflex zones of the feet corresponding
to the abdominal organs

for example, would only cause the intestines to overwork, which will create unpleasant spasms and contractions.

A daily session is a good rhythm to follow, but two sessions a day—one in the morning and the other in the evening—makes it possible to increase the therapeutic effectiveness of the massage. Several weeks of foot massage will be necessary to achieve profound effects.

The same method can be applied to the reflex zone for the liver by those for whom a sluggish liver is a factor in, or the sole reason for, their constipation.

THE QUESTION OF POSITION

Modern human beings evacuate their stools by sitting on a toilet. Our early ancestors, to the contrary, squatted on their heels. The squatting position is a difficult one for modern people to maintain, as we are long out of the habit of squatting. This position, which a person adopts naturally when using a Turkish toilet (a toilet without a bowl) is, however, much more physiologically appropriate. It even strongly encourages evacuation of the bowels.

The squatting position relaxes the muscles of the anal sphincter, encouraging the sphincter to open. It also puts the bottom of the colon into a vertical position, rather than the oblique position the colon assumes when sitting. This facilitates the emptying of the colon's contents. Furthermore, thanks to the compression of the intestinal mass that is caused by squatting, the push made by the abdominal muscles is more effective.

The idea is not to throw away the system of using toilet bowls, but to modify your position when sitting on one, if necessary, to make it more physiologically favorable. This consists of raising your feet by four to eight inches with the help of a stool while sitting on the toilet. For those people whose constipation is not too debilitating, placing their knees in this raised position is sometimes all that is needed to enjoy a proper evacuation.

8 Intestinal Flora and Constipation

The role of the digestive tract is to break the foods ingested into smaller and smaller particles. This work is performed by the enzymes contained in the digestive juices, but also by the microorganisms that make up the intestinal flora. In addition to the chemical decomposition of food molecules by digestive enzymes, food is also broken down thanks to these living organisms, the intestinal microbes.

Intestinal flora is made up of bacteria, bacilli, yeasts, and fungi. Approximately five hundred species of different germs are rubbing shoulders together here. By themselves they form a population of 100 trillion individuals, a number that is greater than the number of cells in the body! As a living organism, each member of this population needs to eat in order to survive. The foods that provide them nourishment are the foods they find in their environment—in other words, the foods that we eat.

Intestinal germs attack the residues of the foods that the digestive juices did not manage to digest or could not fully digest because they were too large. In so doing they liberate useful nutrients:

carbohydrates, proteins, and vitamins. In this way, thanks to the activity of the intestinal flora, everything that enters the intestine is eventually broken down into extremely tiny particles. The result of this work is that the stools become homogenous, uniformly moistened, soft in consistency, and thereby easy to eliminate.

Let's now take a more detailed look at the intestinal flora. It is composed of two major categories of bacteria that occupy definite regions of the small intestine and colon.

THE TWO MAJOR CATEGORIES OF INTESTINAL BACTERIA

The first category consists of bacteria of fermentation and the second contains the bacteria of putrefaction. Their names reveal how each group functions.

The Bacteria of Fermentation

These bacteria initiate the fermentation processes needed to divide food particles. These processes primarily take place on the long molecular chains of carbohydrates, such as starch, but also on the rough fibers of grains (cellulose) and the softer fibers of fruits and vegetables (pectin, inulin). The secretions of the stomach and the liver are not enough to break down these fibers to release their nutrients. Consequently, they reach the intestinal level still intact, and it is the bacteria of fermentation that ensure they will undergo their final transformations.

The greatest number of the fermenting germs are the acidophilus lacto-bacteria and bifidus, which include a number of varieties. They are present in the small intestine and in the ascending and transverse colons. The greatest concentration of these bacteria are found where the small intestine ends and the colon begins, which is to say at the cecum and ascending colon.

The substances produced by fermentation are acidic: lactic acids; acetic acids; propionic acids; and butyric, succinic, and carbonic acids. The consequence of their presence is a slight acidification of the parts of the intestine where they reside.

They acquire a pH of 6 to 6.8, which encourages the survival and evolution of more bacteria of fermentation. Another fortunate consequence of the presence of acids is that they stimulate intestinal peristalsis.

The Bacteria of Putrefaction
The decomposition of the foods for which these bacteria are responsible takes place through putrefaction. They attack undigested food particles, primarily those that are rich in proteins, such as meat, fish, and cheese. Over the course of this process, the proteins that remain in the food debris are divided into

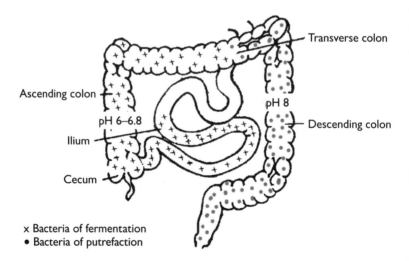

The bacteria of fermentation are found in the small intestine and the ascending and transverse colons; the bacteria of putrefaction are found at the end of the transverse colon and in the descending colon.

short chains of amino acids, then into isolated amino acids.

The principal bacteria of the putrefaction flora belong to the family of the *Escherichia coli* (*E. coli*), of which more than two thousand different species inhabit the colon. Their presence starts at the end of the transverse colon and continues down into the descending colon, an organ in which they are the most numerous.

The putrefaction of proteins produces alkaline substances such as ammonia, phenols, indoles, scatoles, and methane. These substances make the descending colon alkaline in nature (pH 8), which encourages the survival and multiplication of these putrefying bacteria. When the intestinal flora is healthy, the colon has no problem with the production of methane. But when the intestinal flora is imbalanced, this is no longer the case; instead, the production of methane increases. Based on a variety of studies, this substance is presumed to have a hindering effect on intestinal peristalsis.

IMBALANCES OF THE INTESTINAL FLORA

Normally, the intestinal flora is composed of 85 percent bacteria of fermentation and 15 percent bacteria of putrefaction. The proportional difference can be explained by the fact that the bacteria of fermentation colonize a much larger portion of the intestines than the bacteria of putrefaction: 5 meters of the small intestine and 1 meter of the colon for the fermenting bacteria against 50 centimeters of the descending colon for the bacteria of putrefaction.

Nonetheless, we speak of a balance between the two floras when each occupies its part of the intestines without invading the territory of the other. When these conditions prevail, the intestinal flora is described as healthy. It guarantees a good transformation of the alimentary bolus, and then the fecal bolus.

Unfortunately, the bacteria of fermentation and putrefaction do not always maintain these ideal proportions. The size of their respective populations depends on what kinds of foods we eat, as that is their nourishment as well. Population size increases when they receive an abundance of their corresponding foods, but the population shrinks when these foods are not provided. It so happens that in our world today, the diet that is followed by a significant proportion of the population is deficient in grains, fruits, and vegetables, and is therefore poor in the fibers necessary for the development of the bacteria of fermentation. This germ population will therefore shrink in number. The current diet, on the other hand, is rich in meat, cheese, and other proteins, which are favorable for the bacteria of putrefaction, the consequence of which is that the population of this germ increases in size. When they begin to experience tight quarters in the descending colon, the flora of putrefaction begin to colonize the transverse colon and the ascending colon, spreading into a zone of the colon where they should not be. This can happen all the more easily as the flora of fermentation, reduced and anemic, cannot oppose their advance.

This imbalance can sometimes be so significant that the proportions of the two different floras is actually reversed. The flora of fermentation is reduced to 15 percent while the flora of putrefaction swells to 85 percent. An imbalance this significant cannot help but result in negative effects.

INTESTINAL FLORA IMBALANCE AND CONSTIPATION

The negative effects of the imbalance of the intestinal flora on the elimination of stools are many.

A deficiency of intestinal flora will weaken the digestive

process. If good digestion makes good stools, as we have seen, it stands to reason that poor digestion will produce poor stools, which is to say, stools that are hard to evacuate.

Furthermore, the reduction in the number of the bacteria of fermentation automatically creates a reduction in the presence of acids, lactic acids among others. As we have just discussed, these acids stimulate intestinal peristalsis. A reduction in their number therefore leads to a slowdown in transit, which encourages constipation. In addition, when the decreased number of fermentation bacteria results from an insufficient supply of food fiber, the colon is also being deprived of the roughage it needs to function properly.

Meanwhile, the increased population of the bacteria of putrefaction creates a surplus production of alkaline wastes, including methane. The properties of this substance have a hindering effect on intestinal peristalsis, and therefore on the progression of stools through the intestines.

The transverse colon has the ability to perform alternating

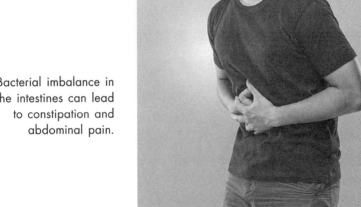

Bacterial imbalance in the intestines can lead to constipation and abdominal pain.

peristaltic movements, both forward and backward, on a portion of its trajectory, in order to hold the fecal bolus at its level. This permits the transverse colon to work the food remnants until they have acquired the characteristics necessary to form good stools. However, when the flora of fermentation is weakened, the transverse colon finds this task quite difficult to perform. Because the fecal bolus is not ready to be sent on into the descending colon, it remains in the transverse colon. By being held there longer than it should, it starts to stagnate there, and thus encourages constipation.

When there is an imbalance of the intestinal flora, the stools will contain poorly digested food residues of various sizes, some of which will be fairly large and more or less hard. The assemblage of these very different kinds of residues does not produce good stools. They will not be moistened uniformly and some parts of them will be too dry. The stools lack consistency, which makes them harder to eliminate. Furthermore, when undigested food remnants that are too large remain in the stools, they have an irritating effect on the mucous membranes of the colon. This causes spasms in the intestinal walls that in turn impede peristaltic movements, and therefore the evacuation of the stools.

PRACTICAL SOLUTIONS

HOW IS THE PROPER BALANCE OF THE INTESTINAL FLORA RESTORED?

An imbalance of the intestinal flora is often present during constipation. Whether this imbalance is large or small, correcting it will support the work of the colon by encouraging the transit and elimination of stools.

Given the fact that the population size of fermenting bacteria and putrefying bacteria depends a great deal on the kinds of food each has at its disposal, a change in diet is imperative as the first corrective measure in remedying constipation.

By reducing the supply of proteins, especially meat proteins, you deprive the bacteria of putrefaction their nourishment. They will weaken, multiplying in lesser numbers and dying off to a certain extent, which will reduce their population. With this loss in numbers, they will have a more difficult time remaining in those parts of the colon that were not theirs originally—the transverse colon and ascending colon. This difficulty will increase if measures for increasing the population of the fermentation bacteria are taken, which will place the two flora in competition with one another. The flora that encourages fermentation will have the upper hand when they are no longer outnumbered, as they are naturally at home in transverse and ascending colons and will find it easy to reoccupy them. This will further force the weakened germs of putrefaction to retreat to their natural habitat in the descending colon.

The repair of the intestinal flora is primarily achieved, therefore, by regenerating the flora of fermentation, given the fact that the healthier it is, the better it can stand up to invasions from the flora of putrefaction.

Two different approaches, which can be employed in combination, are used to regenerate the flora of fermentation. The first consists of properly nourishing these germs by virtue of consuming high-fiber foods, called prebiotics. Being strengthened this way, they multiply more easily and gradually win back their proper place. This is a slow process that occurs over time. However, a person may feel a need to proceed in a more intensive manner. This is where the second approach comes in. It consists of supplying a large number of already existing, living fermentation flora that will immediately be able to become established and get to work in the intestines. The foods or preparations used for this purpose are called probiotics.

THE PREBIOTICS

Origin	Forms	Source
Plant	Fiber	Fruits, vegetables, grains
Animal	Lactose	Whey, lactose (milk) sugar

The consumption of foods rich in fiber (see chapter 3) makes it possible to strengthen the flora of fermentation. These foods, exclusively of plant origin, are fruits, vegetables, and whole grains. Their increase in your diet must be substantial. For your noon or evening meal you might consume a large green salad or a large plate of raw vegetables (carrots, beets, fennel root, cabbage, and so forth) seasoned with cold-pressed virgin oil. In addition, it would be a good idea to introduce one or two generous quantities of cooked vegetables to your meals. Complete grains, in the form of a dish of rice, barley, polenta, buckwheat, or whole grain pasta, for example, should also become a regular part of your meals. Whole grain bread or whole grain breakfast cereals can become a part of your everyday breakfast. Fresh or dried fruits should preferably be eaten between meals as snacks.

These foods that encourage the flourishing of the fermentation bacteria are called prebiotics because they precede (pre) the living (bio), and thus should be supplied to the intestinal bacteria so that they may live. These foods can be rich in either soluble or nonsoluble fibers. In this way, they form not only a fundamental supply of fiber, serving as roughage for filling the intestines and stimulating intestinal peristalsis, but they also supply fiber to nourish the flora of fermentation. Eating roughage, which is so often recommended for fighting constipation, therefore takes action in two ways.

Prebiotics are the fiber on which the flora
of fermentation feeds.

Although prebiotics are primarily of plant origin, some are of animal origin; these come in the form of milk sugar, or lactose. This disaccharide is composed of a glucose molecule and a galactose molecule (*gala* is Greek for milk). As its name indicates, the origin of the galactose molecule is milk. The lactose content of milk is 4.7 grams per liter.

Lactose is a food of choice for the bacteria of fermentation. By digesting it they produce lactic acid, which provides a double benefit. On the one hand, lactic acid slightly acidifies the small intestine and the beginning of the colon, which encourages the multiplication of the fermentation bacteria while creating an adverse environment for the bacteria of putrefaction. As well, as mentioned earlier, lactic acid stimulates intestinal peristalsis. Lactose is therefore a key food for fighting constipation, except of course for those people who are allergic to it or who are lactose intolerant, for whom lactose is contraindicated.

As noted above, lactose only makes up 4.7 grams per liter of milk. Given this minimal supply, a person would have to drink a lot of milk to obtain any therapeutic effect on the intestinal flora. However, there are two products manufactured from milk that supply much higher concentrations of lactose.

The first is whey, the liquid part of the curd that appears during the process of making cheese (see chapter 4; for more on whey's benefits, see my book *The Whey Prescription*). Using special processes, it is transformed into powder or flakes. The whey in powder form has a high lactose content—75 percent by volume. Whey powder can be purchased at natural foods stores in plain or flavored varieties. It is mixed with water before ingesting.

Whey

Intensive Cure

Mix 1 or 2 tablespoons of whey powder with water. Drink three to six glasses a day. You must drink the reconstituted whey immediately so that it does not turn rancid.

Be aware that whey has a laxative effect when used in high doses.

Maintenance Dose

One or two glasses of reconstituted whey a day.

Lactose (Milk) Sugar

Lactose can be extracted from whey. The concentrate obtained this way is sold under the name lactose or milk sugar. It is 100 percent lactose. When mixed with water this powder produces a beverage with a pleasant and slightly sweet flavor. Milk sugar powder can also be used by mixing it in with various foods such as yogurts or desserts.

Milk sugar supports the flora of fermentation and helps it develop. It also stimulates intestinal transit by slightly acidifying the small intestine. The disappearance of the bloating that accompanies this regimen is evidence of the beneficial action of lactose on the intestinal flora.

Intensive Cure

Mix 1 tablespoon of lactose with water, or with plain yogurt with bifidus cultures. Drink three times a day.

Maintenance Dose

1 tablespoon of lactose a day.

Whey and lactose sugar are supplements for the diet. They can be used as a therapeutic regimen for one or two months, or more if needed. These regimens must be regularly renewed by people who are subject to chronic imbalances in the intestinal flora.

On the other hand, the prebiotics that are fruits, vegetables, and grains all form part of what nature has planned for our intestines and should consequently be eaten on a daily basis for your entire life.

PROBIOTICS

Probiotic preparations, which are employed to rapidly seed the intestines, prove most effective under specific conditions. The bacteria used must be fermentation flora. They should also be habitual guests of the intestines. This is essential so that they can survive there. Using foreign and non-adapted bacteria makes no sense, as they will not be able to withstand their environment and will rapidly die. The probiotic bacteria should be living and able to remain that way until they reach the intestines. The extremely acidic pH of the stomach has a destructive effect on bacteria. When freeze-dried bacteria are used, they must be a kind that can reanimate.

> Probiotic preparations are used to rapidly seed the intestines with fermentation bacteria.

Freeze drying is a process in which germs are delicately dehydrated and dried. This drying process does not kill the bacteria but renders them momentarily inactive. They will come out of their forced slumber when they enter the moist, warm environment of the intestines. Rehydrated and reactivated, they will settle in and start developing in their new home.

There are three kinds of probiotics.

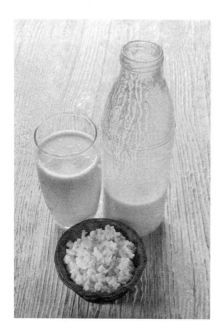

Probiotic preparations

Probiotic Yogurts

Milk is transformed into yogurt by the bacteria of fermentation it contains that cause the milk to curdle. These bacteria that are necessary for the manufacture of yogurt are added to it and remain in the finished product. People who eat yogurt will thereby help their intestinal flora, but only if the bacteria culture is alive. It so happens that the high temperatures used in the manufacture of yogurt tends to kill these germs. Such yogurts therefore offer no beneficial effects for the intestinal flora.

However, some yogurts are manufactured specifically for the bacteria to survive, so the bacteria can live and in turn help the intestines. Yogurts created this way, by only slightly heating the milk, are called probiotics because they are good (pro) for life (bio). The bacteria are able to withstand the acidity of the gastric secretions with no great problem. They have been selected among the normal guests of the intestines because they are able to establish themselves easily there. These bacteria are lactobacillus acidophilus and bifidus.

Good to Know

It is preferable to consume plain yogurts to avoid taking in too much white sugar. If necessary, plain yogurt can be sweetened with whole, unrefined sugar.

Intensive Cure

Eat three to five servings of probiotic yogurt (with bifidus or acidophilus cultures or both) over the course of the day.

Maintenance Dose

Eat one serving of probiotic yogurt a day.

Active Concentrates

The preparation of these concentrates is similar to that of yogurt, but the final product is a bit more concentrated. Concentrates are sold in small bottles (usually about 100 ml), often bearing a name that starts with the prefix "acti"; for example, Actimel, also known as DanActive, produced by Dannon. Yakult also makes a probiotic drink. A rapid reseeding of the intestines can be achieved in several weeks by ingesting two to three of these bottles a day.

Intensive Cure

Drink 2 to 3 bottles a day.

Maintenance Dose

Drink 1 bottle a day.

Laboratory Preparations

The concentration of bacteria in these products is generally higher than that of the two products discussed above. The freeze-dried bacteria comes back to life once it has entered the intestines. These preparations are shaped in the form of tablets or sold as a powder to mix with liquid.

For directions on using these products, consult the manufacturer's instructions.

PROBIOTIC PREPARATIONS

Country of Origin	Product Name	Producer
United States	SureBiotics	M2 Products Group
	Complete Probiotics	Mercola
	Bactipro	Medix Select
	Probiotic Defense	NOW Foods
	RAW Probiotics	Garden of Life
	Ultimate Flora	Renew Life
Canada	Probiotic capsules	Bio-K Plus
	Probaclac	Nicar Labs
France	Florastor	Biocodex
	Acidophylus/Bifidus	Vit'all
	Bifido Factor	Natren
	Lactibiane	Pileje
	Entéroflore	Laboratoires Yves Ponroy
	Ergyphilus	Laboratoire Nutergia
Belgium	Bifibiol	Bio-Life
	Proflor Plus	PharmaNutrics
	Aadexil	Springfield
Switzerland	Bioflorin	Sanofi-Aventis
	Lactoferment 5/10	Axcan Pharma

9 Nerves, Stress, and Constipation

The functioning of the intestines is organized and administered by the nervous system.

The walls of the intestines are carpeted with very sensitive nerves. They record the distension of the walls caused by the arrival of food. They then send a signal to the motor nerves that control the peristaltic muscles. These nerves are controlled by the autonomic nervous system, which can accelerate or slow down intestinal function, depending on the body's needs.

Like any other organ, under normal circumstances the nervous system is more or less strong and enjoys good health. However, emotions, fears, and worries can have an influence on how it functions. When the nervous system's functioning has been disrupted, it helps constipation to become established.

THE INFLUENCE OF THE AUTONOMIC NERVOUS SYSTEM

The function of all the organs in the body is under the management of the autonomic nervous system. As indicated by its name, it is autonomous, which means it is not subject to our will but functions independently of our desires. It regulates and coordinates all organic functions without our having to do anything, or to even think about it. The autonomic nervous system oversees the adaptation of our glandular and organ function to meet the needs of our body. Its purpose is to ensure our body is at its best—which is to say that we are in a state of full health.

The autonomic nervous system is made up of two separate subsystems with opposing functions: the sympathetic nervous system and the parasympathetic nervous system.

The sympathetic nervous system increases the tone of the organs and the strength of muscular contractions, and it accelerates the work of the organs. On the intestinal level this means that the sympathetic nervous system sees to it that the peristaltic muscles will always enjoy better tone, contract with greater intensity, and work at a more sustainable rhythm, ensuring an acceleration of the work performed by the digestive tract.

The parasympathetic nervous system has an opposite function. It reduces the tone of the organs, the strength of muscular contractions, and the work rhythm of the organs. The effect of the parasympathetic system on the intestines ensures that the peristaltic muscles have less tone, Their contractions will be weaker and occur at a slower rhythm, resulting in the work of the intestines slowing down.

The sympathetic and parasympathetic nervous systems work in close collaboration. At any given moment one of these systems will be dominant; then, based on the needs of the body, the other one will get the upper hand. In this way the organs are stimulated and slowed down in such a way to always be in a position to meet the body's needs. A continual adaptation to new situations and demands takes place. If nothing happens to impede this harmonious collaboration, the body will function at its best.

Stress can throw the autonomic nervous system out of whack, however. Its effect will be exhibited differently on the sympathetic and parasympathetic functions.

Stress pushes the sympathetic nervous system to function even more intensely. It further reinforces the tone, strength, and

PARASYMPATHETIC NERVOUS SYSTEM   SYMPATHETIC NERVOUS SYSTEM

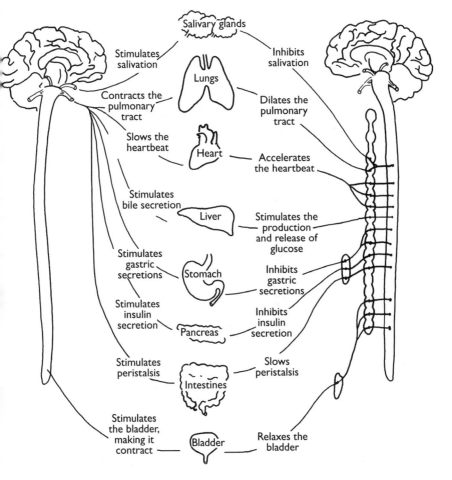

The two aspects of the nervous system and their functions

rhythm of muscular contractions. In the intestines, this causes an acceleration of intestinal functions that cause diarrhea. One of the most common examples in which this occurs is in the experience of stage fright. For some people, the intensified muscular contractions will even cause spasms and intestinal blockages, which in turn cause constipation.

The effect of stress on the parasympathetic nervous system is different but also leads to constipation. Stress increases the relaxation and loosening of intestinal function. The peristaltic muscles lose their tone and become too passive, soft, and slow. Constipation becomes established. The function of the parasympathetic nervous system is, in fact, to slow things down. When it is stimulated, it does not push the intestines to behave more actively but instead to behave more slowly.

For some people, the disruption of the autonomic nervous system by stress is the sole cause of constipation. For others stress is only an aggravating factor, and the primary cause of constipation is something else. In either case, however, it is a good idea to learn how to manage stress in a way that it does not impede the functioning of the autonomic nervous system. The best means for controlling stress is learning how to control your breathing and to relax.

BREATH CONTROL

It was noted earlier that the physiological functions governed by the autonomic nervous system are not subject to our direct control. But this is not quite true. There is a function under our control that can affect the autonomic nervous system—that is the respiratory function. Through directed effort we can slow or accelerate our breathing. This ability to control our breathing is an extremely valuable strategy for calming ourselves by slowing the rate of our inhalations and exhalations. By intentionally slowing the rhythm of our breathing, we also slow the rhythm of the heart. As it happens, the heart not only reacts strongly to the emotions that stress arouses, but the rhythm of our heartbeat influences that of the other organs.

A person who is feeling stressed is unable to slow his or her cardiac rhythm and lower his or her blood pressure in order to restore a feeling of calm. The cardiac function, in fact, is not something a person can control directly. On the other hand, he or she can work on it indirectly by means of respiration. This is how a person can free him- or herself from the negative effects of stress.

To learn how to control your breathing it is necessary to breathe into your belly with the help of the diaphragm, an umbrella-shaped muscle located at the base of the lungs.

PRACTICAL SOLUTIONS
CONTROLLING YOUR BREATHING

- Lie flat on your back on a bed or on the ground.
- Place your hands on the hollow of your stomach—the location of the diaphragm.
- Exhale slowly while monitoring your diaphragm in order to empty your lungs, which amounts to intentionally sucking in your abdomen. The diaphragm will be pushed up and exert pressure on the lungs, forcing them to empty themselves of their content.
- Once the lungs are empty, inhale slowly and push the diaphragm downward. By moving away from the lungs the diaphragm frees them, thereby allowing the incoming air to penetrate them more abundantly.

This breathing exercise should be repeated a dozen times in a row, two times a day. Over time you will master the technique of breathing through the diaphragm and will be able to employ it when standing up.

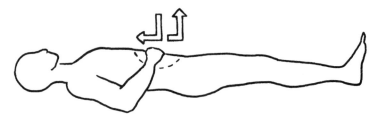

Practice diaphragmatic breathing to slow the breathing rhythm and increase the oxygen intake.

Breath control not only consists of breathing more deeply but also of slowing the rhythm at which you are breathing. In the beginning, force yourself to slow down by counting to 5 when exhaling and to 5 when inhaling. With habit, the length of inhalation and exhalation can be gradually increased by counting to 6, 7, 8, 9, and so forth. The rate of respiration can be slowed even further by taking a brief pause of one to two seconds between inhaling and exhaling.

Good to Know

These exercises can also be performed while walking.

Practice controlling your breathing the next time a stressful situation arises. As soon as you are aware that a sensation of stress is starting—in other words, when you feel as if everything in you is racing, whether it's your physical body or your thoughts and emotions, take a deep breath, then impose a slower rhythm on your breathing.

RELAXATION PRACTICE

The effect of stress on the sympathetic nervous system is felt on the muscular level as it causes your muscles to contract. They will feel strained and taut for no reason. These muscular contractions create a state of tension that can irritate and annoy a person, thereby increasing his or her initial stress. This rise in the level of stress can be combated by actively relaxing.

> Relaxation is a technique aiming to intentionally loosen all
> the muscles in your body for the purpose of
> helping you get looser emotionally.

- Lie on your back on a bed or on the ground.
- Become aware of your feet and relax them, changing their position if necessary.
- Now become aware of your calves. Are your calves relaxed or not? If they are not, relax them.
- Proceed in the same manner, rising from one part of your body to the next: from thighs to buttocks to hips.
- Next move to the hands, arms, and shoulders.
- To end, move to the back, the nape of the neck, and the head, including the eyes and the jaw.
- Check to see if your entire body is relaxed by mentally scanning all these parts again in the same order as before.
- Once you are completely relaxed, slow your breathing rhythm using the diaphragmatic breathing method presented above.
- Focus your attention on the air that enters and leaves your lungs for five to ten minutes, depending on your needs.

With habit, you will soon be able to relax your body quickly and easily. Occasions to practice a relaxation session are obviously rare when you're in the middle of a stressful situation, at work or anywhere else. But by doing this regularly, once or twice a day, you will increase your own resistance to stress, making it possible to approach stressful situations by being more relaxed and allowing you to recover more quickly afterward. Over the long term your entire body will benefit, and your intestines will as well. They will cease being regularly blocked by stress and can return to their proper function.

10 Nutritional Deficiencies and Constipation

Deficiencies in nutrients such as vitamins and minerals can lead to poor intestinal function. These deficiencies are not a primary cause of constipation, but they can contribute to it.

Every organ requires nutrients to function and regenerate, and

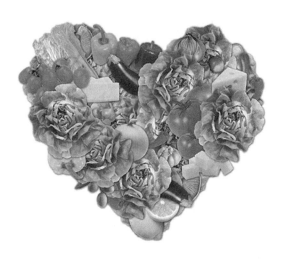

Sufficient nutrients such as vitamins and minerals in the diet contribute to intestinal health.

the intestines are no exception. Nutrients are essential for the development and repair of organic tissues, the production of energy, the manufacture of secretions, the transmission of nerve signals, and the contraction of the muscles.

When the intestines receive all the nutrients they need, the peristaltic and eliminatory muscles are well toned and developed, the nerves are powerfully reactive, and intestines' mucous glands can produce generous secretions. These characteristics are the exact opposite of those that typify the intestines of a constipated person: sluggish and poorly toned muscles, weak nerves that have great difficulty reacting, miserly secretions of mucus, and so forth.

Good nutrition is therefore essential in the fight against intestinal laziness. So just what role do the various nutrients play in the functioning of the intestines?

NUTRIENTS AND THEIR EFFECT ON THE INTESTINES

Proteins

Proteins are the building blocks that the muscles use to build and repair themselves. Muscles require proteins in order to develop, to become large and strong.

Deficiency

A lack of protein will lead to atrophy and sluggishness of the abdominal, peristaltic, and eliminatory muscles.

Source

Animal proteins, such as meat, fish, eggs, and cheese, are a more certain and generous source of proteins than those of plant origin: beans, grains, and oleaginous foods.

Vitamin A

Vitamin A is active in the regeneration of the intestinal mucous membranes. It ensures that the membranes remain flexible and well lubricated.

Deficiency

When vitamin A is deficient, the mucous membranes will start to dry out. They are not as well protected as they should be due to this lack of mucus, and therefore the walls are not slippery enough to ensure the easy passage of stools.

Source

The animal sources of vitamin A are eggs and, most especially, halibut and cod liver oils, which can be bought as dietary supplements. The plant foods that are rich in vitamin A are carrots, squash, cabbage, spinach, and green vegetables in general, as well as apricots, melon, and tomatoes.

B Vitamins

There are about fifteen different vitamins included in the vitamin B complex. They are most often combined in the same foods and work in close synergy with each other.

B vitamins actively contribute to the production of energy. They are therefore the vitamins that ensure that the peristaltic muscles will have the energy required to function properly. They also contribute significantly to ensuring that the sensitive nerves of the mucous membranes will be strong and capable of clearly transmitting their impulses to the muscles of the intestines.

Deficiency

The lack of B-complex vitamins makes the intestinal muscles and nerves weak, lazy, and slow to react.

Source

The main sources for B vitamins are whole grains, wheat germ, and brewer's yeast.

Vitamin C

Vitamin C is necessary for the growth of tissue and the mucous membranes. It also maintains the rhythm of organ activity.

Deficiency

The lack of vitamin C in your diet will lead to a weakening of the intestinal muscles and a slowing of intestinal peristalsis.

Source

The principal sources of vitamin C are fruits in general, but especially the citrus fruits, kiwi, black currant, and strawberries. While all raw vegetables contain vitamin C, green and red peppers, cabbage, spinach, parsley, and broccoli are especially high in this vitamin.

Vitamin E

Vitamin E provides good tone to the intestinal muscles and helps keep the mucous membranes flexible and lubricated.

Deficiency

A lack of vitamin E will cause the peristaltic and eliminatory muscles to become weak and slow to react. The intestinal mucous membranes dry out and become less slippery.

Source

The sources of vitamin E are whole grains, wheat germ, cold-pressed virgin oils (sunflower, walnut, and grapeseed), and oleaginous fruits. Wheat germ is especially high in vitamin E.

Omegas 3, 6 (Vitamin F)

Omega-3s and omega-6s work together in the building of the mucous membranes. They give the membranes resistance and flexibility by encouraging the release of lubricating mucus.

Deficiency

Without the omegas in your diet, the intestinal mucous membranes dry out and become porous. They can then allow toxins to enter the bloodstream.

Source

Omega-3s and omega-6s are found in cold-pressed virgin plant oils—flax, safflower, canola, soy, and sunflower, to name a few—and in oleaginous fruits—nuts and seeds.

Calcium

Calcium encourages the progression of nerve impulse along the nerves and thereby encourages stimulation of the peristaltic muscles.

Deficiency

When a calcium deficiency exists, the nerves will not react as well as they should, and muscles will either contract poorly or too much (spasms).

Source

The primary source of calcium is dairy products. Sardines and salmon are also rich in this mineral. Some other foods, such as carrots, green vegetables, and almonds, also contain calcium, but in smaller amounts.

Iron

Iron is necessary to ensure that the cells get a sufficient supply of oxygen, which determines the strength with which the muscles can act.

Deficiency

In the event of an iron deficiency, the intestinal muscles will be weak due to under-oxygenation.

Source

Iron can be found in whole grains, spinach, red beets, apricots, carrots, cabbage, and eggs.

Magnesium

Magnesium is a necessary nutrient for the good functioning of nerves and muscles, giving them tone and vigor.

Deficiency

When there is a lack of magnesium in the body, the nerves will be weak and their impulses will be transmitted poorly. Muscular contraction will be insufficient, which will cause a slowdown of intestinal transit and sometimes cause cramps or spasms.

Source

Foods that are rich in magnesium include whole grains, oleaginous foods, and green vegetables, as well as seafood.

Potassium

This mineral is essential for proper muscular contraction and for the transmission of nerve impulses.

Deficiency

When there is a lack of potassium in the body, the intestinal and eliminatory muscles will perform poorly. Another problem caused by lack of potassium is that the nerve impulses sent from the intestine's sensitive nerves will be reduced.

Source

Potassium is abundant in fruits and vegetables.

Sulfur

Sulfur is a mineral that is essential for the liver. This is how sulfur contributes indirectly to good intestinal function.

Deficiency

A sulfur deficiency leads to intestinal laziness due to a lack of bile.

Source

Sulfur can be found in animal meats and eggs, as well as in sulfured vegetables such as leeks, onions, garlic, radish, turnip, asparagus, watercress, and cabbage.

PRACTICAL SOLUTIONS

HOW TO FILL NUTRITIONAL DEFICIENCIES

Deficiencies appear when a person is not eating enough, or any, of certain foods that form the basic healthy human diet. In fact, all the nutrients the body needs can be found in the bounty of foods offered us by nature. A person suffering from a nutritional deficiency must reintroduce the appropriate foods into his or her diet, to address the deficiencies over time.

The sources of the various nutrients listed above show that a vast portion of them are supplied by fruits, vegetables, and whole grains. However, these foods are also the ones that are high in fiber. A constipated person who changes her diet in order to consume more roughage will also, over time, rectify a large part of her nutritional deficiencies. As a general rule, this dietary intervention is enough, but in some cases the deficiencies are too deep and a more energetic intervention is called for: taking nutritional concentrates in the form of natural dietary supplements.

Natural dietary supplements are concentrates of the amino acids, vitamins, and minerals offered by nature. Their nutrients are easy to assimilate because of their concentration, and they fill any deficiencies much more quickly. The variety of nutrients that are available in this form ensures that any nutrients a person may be lacking can be sufficiently addressed. Indeed, it is not always easy to determine exactly which nutrients we may be lacking.

There are many different kinds of natural food supplements, but some are especially valuable in the battle against constipation.

Bee Pollen

This is the flower pollen that has been collected by bees and brought to the hive in the form of small pellets stuck to their legs. Bee pollen is made up of 35 percent protein and includes the eight amino acids essential for human beings. It is extremely high in methionine (3.5 grams per 100 grams), which the liver particularly needs. As we know, a strong liver encourages good intestinal functioning by virtue of the bile it secretes. Pollen contains all the existing vitamins except two: vitamin F and vitamin B4. Its high vitamin C content (6 grams per 100 grams) ramps up intestinal function, and its B vitamins supply the energy that the peristaltic muscles need. These muscles are also toned by the vitamin E found in bee pollen, as well as by the potassium, calcium, iron, and magnesium it contains.

In addition to its nutritive virtues, bee pollen has proven to be a gentle and effective intestinal stimulant.

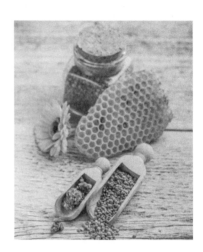

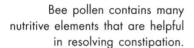
Bee pollen contains many nutritive elements that are helpful in resolving constipation.

Therapeutic Regimen

1 teaspoon of bee pollen pellets a day, diluted in a drink or blended with yogurt. It should be ingested every morning for one to three months.

Contraindications

Bee pollen is contraindicated for people with heart problems and those with high blood pressure.

Good to Know

Some people who take bee pollen will experience a very stimulating effect to their heart and nerves.

Blackstrap Molasses

Blackstrap molasses is a by-product of the extraction of sugar from sugarcane. It is extremely high in minerals; in fact, several minerals are present in molasses at record rates, including potassium (1.9 to 3.3 grams per 100 grams), calcium (0.8 to 1.4 grams per 100 grams), and magnesium (0.2 grams to 0.4 grams per 100 grams).

These minerals are all necessary for good muscle function and nerve function in the intestines. Moreover, their action is supported by the presence of vitamins A and B.

In addition, through its overall composition, blackstrap molasses has demonstrated laxative properties when taken in sufficient doses.

Therapeutic Regimen

2 to 3 teaspoons of blackstrap molasses a day stirred into warm water. Drink it in small sips, to which you incorporate a healthy amount of saliva. The duration of the therapeutic regimen can be from two to three months.

Brewer's Yeast

Brewer's yeast is a microscopic fungus used in the brewing of beer. Brewer's yeast is extremely rich in B vitamins. Not only are all the vitamins of this complex present, but they are present in very high concentrations. The B vitamins are essential for the production of energy, which includes the energy the peristaltic muscles require to function properly. Its stimulating and toning action on the intestines is also explained by its high content of the essential amino acids required by the muscles, and by the presence of various minerals, including magnesium and potassium, which encourage good transmission of nerve impulses.

Therapeutic Regimen

The yeasts to use for this purpose are the yeasts used for beer or food. They can come in the form of flakes or powder, or even as tablets. The dose is 1 heaping tablespoon (around 14 grams) a day to be sprinkled over cooked foods or mixed with yogurt or salad dressing. The dose for tablets depends on their size, so it is necessary to check the manufacturer's instructions. A therapeutic regimen can last from one to three months, as needed.

Contraindication
Brewer's yeast is not advised for people suffering from candida.

Seaweed
Kelp and bladder wrack are two kinds of seaweed that are used as food supplements. They are rich in mineral salts, particularly potassium, calcium, magnesium, sulfur, iron, and iodine. In fact, seaweeds contain all the minerals in existence, thus they have a stimulating effect on the body overall when ingested, particularly on the intestines. Seaweeds are especially recommended for constipated individuals who are fatigued, who lack tone in general, and whose metabolisms are working too slowly.

Therapeutic Regimen
Taking seaweed in the form of tablets or gel caps is the simplest way to follow a therapeutic regimen. Follow the instructions provided by the manufacturer.

Contraindications
Seaweed is contraindicated for people who are nervous, easily excited, stressed, and/or suffering from hyperthyroid issues.

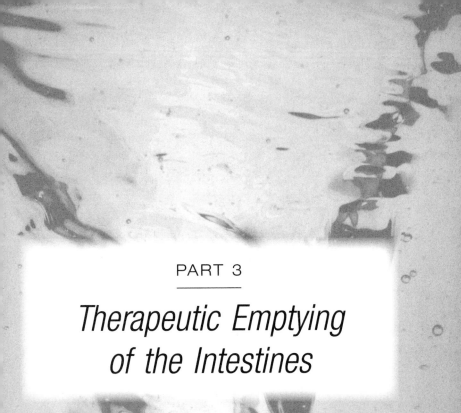

PART 3

Therapeutic Emptying of the Intestines

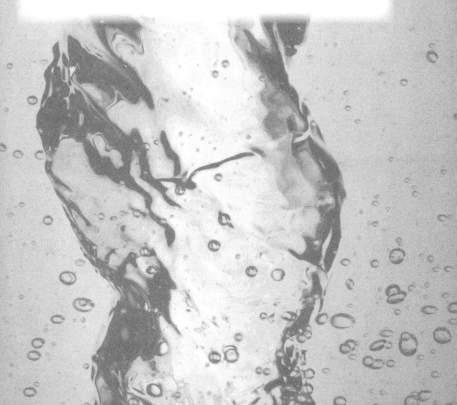

11 Laxatives, Purges, and Enemas

The hygienic measures introduced in part 2 of this book—eating more roughage, increasing fluid consumption, toning the abdominal muscles, and so forth—are sufficient in the majority of cases to restore a normal intestinal transit.

In other cases, though, the intestines have been weakened and become lazy, and these measures will not be enough to restore proper function. The continued accumulation of matter is hampering their ability to perform. The intestines are filled with too much material, which is stagnating and causing congestion in the colon. An energetic intervention from the outside is therefore essential for liberating the intestines. By artificially draining them, you will unblock them. At the same time, this is an opportunity to put them back into proper working order, which is not possible when they are overburdened with wastes. The means used for this purpose do not fall into the domain of hygiene—they are to be considered therapeutic, and their use should be time limited.

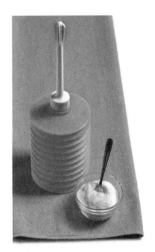

Enemas, purges, and laxatives are sometimes needed to get the intestines moving properly again.

Laxatives, enemas, and purges are valuable aids for short-term fixes, but they are not suitable for addressing constipation long term.

Laxatives, purges, and enemas are effective methods for stimulating the intestines. However, they do not represent a sustainable solution to the problem of constipation. In fact, will the intestines once again function normally once they have been emptied? It is extremely rare for this to ever be the case. These methods do not change the lifestyle choices—the lack of roughage and fluids, weak abdominal muscle tone, and so forth—that are responsible for constipation. Therefore, these methods cannot provide a lasting cure for constipation.

We will examine each of these methods now.

LAXATIVES

Laxatives are remedies that encourage the evacuation of stools. Purges do the same thing, but in a much more violent and rapid way, so much more that they will be looked at in a separate section. Fundamentally, though, the way these two methods work is identical—it is only the intensity with which they work that defines them. Therefore, a laxative used in a higher dosage can turn into a purgative.

Laxatives stimulate intestinal peristalsis. They compel the intestinal muscles to work. The muscles contract more strongly and at a faster rhythm. Mucus secretions increase in quantity. Laxatives also possess the property of making stools more liquid and soft. All these effects contribute to helping stools advance more easily through the colon and encourage their evacuation.

People who take a laxative (or a purgative) for the first time are always astonished by the quantity of stools that are eliminated. This large quantity can be attributed to the fact that it is not only the daily wastes being eliminated, but the waste matter that has collected over time in the colon and formed deposits on its walls.

The ideal dose for a laxative is one that makes it possible to obtain one or two stools a day that are soft enough to be evacuated spontaneously. The correct dose depends on the person and needs to be figured out through trial and error. If the dose is too low, no changes will appear with regard to evacuations. The dose should then be increased gradually from day to day until the desired effect has been obtained. Once the correct dose has been discovered, it is maintained for the duration of the regimen.

If the dose is too high, the stools will become too liquid and too frequent, as is the case with diarrhea. They will exhaust and irritate the intestines. In this case, the advice is not to gradually lower the dosage but to instead stop any laxatives for several days in order to give your colon a chance to rest. When you resume taking laxatives, start with smaller doses or with a gentler laxative.

A perfectly dosed laxative will act gently. It has a slightly rehabilitative effect because it stimulates the colon and helps improve its function. The colon is strengthened and adapts to a new work rhythm. To benefit from these effects, the period of time during which laxatives are taken should be from one to three weeks. It is a good idea to stop the regimen after this span of time to prevent the colon from becoming accustomed to only working under the impetus of laxatives. In fact, the colon should be habituated to function independently using the hygienic measures described in part 2 of this book.

Good to Know

One physiologically based method to interrupt a laxative regimen consists of gradually reducing the dose during the last week of the therapy. In this way the colon becomes used to functioning less and less with the help of laxatives and more and more through its own forces.

There are three major ways of stimulating the colon with laxatives. Some laxatives work primarily on intestinal peristalsis, while others work by increasing the amount of water in the colon. The third method consists of making the intestinal walls more slippery. For this reason, laxatives can be divided into three categories: stimulating, osmotic, and lubricating.

THE THREE KINDS OF LAXATIVES

Name	The Way They Work
Stimulating laxatives	Accelerate intestinal peristalsis
Osmotic laxatives	Draw water into the colon
Lubricating laxatives	Make the intestinal walls slippery

These three categories of laxatives will now be described, along with how they work and the way they are taken.

STIMULATING LAXATIVES

The chemical substances contained in these laxatives have a stimulating effect on intestinal peristalsis. They begin to work once they have made contact with the intestinal mucous membranes, which is the reason they are also called "contact laxatives."

The active properties of these laxatives act on the nerve endings located in the mucous membranes of the colon. This stimulation of the colon nerves causes an intense reaction. This in turn causes strong contractions of the peristaltic muscles. Their reinvigorated activity helps advance stools through the colon. This stimulation by chemical substances also obliges the mucous membranes to secrete more mucus to protect themselves, which lubricates the colon and makes the stools more fluid. This process of increasing the fluid content of the stools is also caused by hydrophilic substances (which attract water and trigger osmotic exchanges) contained in the laxative. The water drawn from the surrounding tissue enters the colon and liquefies the stools. Here are a few plants that are the most commonly used stimulating laxatives.

Alder Buckthorn (Rhamnus frangula)
The bark of this bush, a European native now widespread in rural areas of the United States from Maine to South Dakota, is enthusiastically recommended as a laxative. Its action is gentle and well tolerated by the body.

Gel Caps
1 in the morning and 1 at night.

Mother Tincture
15 to 30 drops three times a day, or 50 drops once in the evening.

Cassia (Cassia fistula)

A gentle laxative that is pleasant to take. The pulp of this fruit can be eaten like candy.

Pulp

3 or more slices of the flesh of this fruit (from inside the pod).

Decoction

50 grams of the crushed pod per ½ deciliter of water. Boil for 10 minutes. Drink one cup in the evening.

Hemp Agrimony (Eupatorium cannabinum)

A gentle and bitter laxative.

Tea

20 grams of leaves per 1 liter of water. Steep for 10 minutes. Drink two to three cups of this bitter-tasting tea a day.

Decoction

1 teaspoon of root per 1 cup of water. Boil for 2 minutes, then steep for 10 minutes. Drink one to two cups a day.

Licorice (Glycyrrhiza glabra)

Among its many properties, licorice is an antispasmodic for the digestive tract and a laxative. One of its advantages that should not be understated is that it is slightly sweet and has a very pleasant taste. For this reason, licorice is often found as an ingredient in many blends.

Decoction

50 grams per 1 liter of water. Boil 5 minutes, then macerate for 12 hours. Drink one or two cups a day.

Gel Caps

1 or 2 gel caps three times a day.

Peach (**Amygdalus persica**)

A gentle laxative recommended for people with low vitality, and for children.

Tea

1 tablespoon of flowers per cup. Steep for 10 minutes. Drink one or two cups a day.

Round Leaf and Common Mallow (**Malva rotundifolia** *et* **sylvestris**)

A gentle, nonirritating laxative. It is recommended in cases of chronic constipation (atonic or spasmodic), and especially when there is inflammation of the digestive tract.

Tea

40 grams of leaves and/or flowers per 1 liter of water. Steep for 10 minutes. Drink one to two cups a day.

Gel Caps

1 or 2 gel caps three times a day.

Mother Tincture

20 to 50 drops three times a day.

OSMOTIC LAXATIVES

As discussed in chapter 4, osmosis is the phenomenon of exchange that takes place between two fluids separated by a permeable membrane. The fluid that is less concentrated gives up its water to the one that is thicker in order to balance the concentration of the two fluids.

The substances contained in osmotic laxatives significantly increase the density of the liquid present in the colon, which triggers a physiological demand for water. This water comes out of the surrounding tissue and enters the colon by crossing through the colon's mucous membranes.

The supply of water obtained this way moistens the stools and softens them. Depending on the dosage of these osmotic laxatives, the presence of their active principles will be more or less elevated, and the demand for water they trigger will be more or less proportionate to their presence.

The softening of the stools provides favorable circumstances for their evacuation. This is further increased by the fact that the weight of the stools, added to that of the water that has entered the colon, exerts a strong pressure that stimulates intestinal peristalsis and the contraction of the rectal muscles necessary to defecate.

There are two kinds of osmotic laxatives: sweetened osmotic laxatives and saline laxatives.

SWEETENED OSMOTIC LAXATIVES

The sugars we are talking about here are those that arrive in their original state in the colon without having been digested higher up in the digestive tract. They are also poorly digested in the colon. Their presence increases the density of the liquid present in the colon and triggers an osmotic transfer that will invite more water into it.

These sugars are lactose, lactitol, and lactulose. We already discussed lactose in regard to whey in chapter 4 and showed its laxative effects when a sufficient dose is taken.

Two sugars of plant origin also possess laxative virtues: sorbitol and mannitol. Sorbitol can be found in dried prunes and other fruits (for more see chapter 4). A laxative effect can be produced by eating enough of these kinds of fruits.

Mannitol is found in the viscous secretions of certain plants, such as that of a particular variety of ash tree, the *Fraxinus ornus* (flowering ash). The sweet exudation from its stems is called manna. Manna is an efficient and gentle laxative. Thanks to its flavor, it is pleasant to take.

Common Polypody (Polypodium vulgare)

Decoction

40 grams per 1 liter of water. Boil for 2 minutes, then allow to steep for 10 minutes. Drink one to two cups a day.

Flowering Ash (Fraxinus ornus)

Drops

5 to 10 grams for a child of fifteen months or younger.
10 to 15 grams up to the age of three.
15 to 20 grams for children between the ages of three and five.
20 to 30 grams for a child over five.
50 to 60 grams for adults.

Take once a day diluted in lukewarm water, preferably in the evening.

Another laxative plant rich in carbohydrates is the common polypody. This is a fern that is widely distributed throughout Europe and whose roots have been used for more than two thousand years to stimulate the intestines. They have a slight licorice flavor, which makes them pleasant to take.

SALINE OSMOTIC LAXATIVES

The composition of saline osmotic laxatives is exclusively mineral. They are comprised of mineral salts such as sodium and potassium, phosphates, and magnesium chloride. As little if any of them are absorbed, these minerals remain in the colon, to which they will draw water through the process of osmosis.

Numerous saline laxatives can be found for sale in the health market in the form of powder, tablets, and gel caps. These laxatives are less natural than plants, as they cannot be found in this state in nature. They are effective, however, and sometimes easier for the body to tolerate. Here are several examples.

Magnesium Chloride
20 grams per liter of water; take 2 to 3 tablespoons, or more, of this blend a day. The dose should be diluted in a glass of water, and preferably taken in the evening.

Milk of Magnesia (**Magnesium hydroxide**)
1 or 2 teaspoons with water. Take at night before going to bed.

THE LUBRICATING LAXATIVES

The lubricating laxatives encourage stools to slip through the colon, thanks to the greasy or oily substances they contain. As they are not absorbed by the body, they are deposited on the walls of the colon and thereby facilitate the evacuation of the stools. Furthermore, because of their presence on the mucous membranes, they reduce the amount of water that is absorbed from the fecal bolus. For this reason it is easier for the stools to retain their optimum moistness and softness.

Glycerin suppositories belong to this category of laxative, but I do not recommend them. They make it possible to produce stools rapidly (in five to twenty minutes), but they are irritants. When used too often they will cause rectal irritations. They can be replaced by rectal douches (see page 171) with much better results.

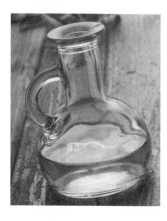

Consuming food-grade oil in the morning on an empty stomach lubricates the intestines.

Virgin Olive Oil

The consumption of food oil in the morning on an empty stomach has a lubricating effect on the intestines.

One part of the oil is in fact not digested and instead makes the stools and colon walls slippery. Any kind of food-grade oil can be used, but the one recommended most often is olive oil. Take 1 to 2 tablespoons of olive oil in the morning, on an empty stomach.

Good to Know

As constipation is such a widespread problem, there are many special preparations available in the marketplace. They combine several elements that encourage the restoration of good intestinal transit and the evacuation of stools. These specialty products combine the benefits of roughage with those of laxative plants and substances that will trigger osmosis. They can be used to one's benefit.

PURGES

A purge, or purgative, acts like a laxative, but in a much more intense way. The stools become very fluid and are quickly eliminated because they stimulate intestinal peristalsis quite strongly.

The procedure is rapid and efficient. The urge to defecate becomes imperative, and evacuation happens of its own accord, almost without the person being able to hold it back. It is therefore violent. The quantities of stools evacuated are also elevated. Purges affect the entire colon.

> With a purge, the stools become very liquid and are abruptly evacuated.

The effectiveness of purges is of benefit in emergency situations, when a person needs to unblock and rapidly empty the colon. But the radical nature of the method is also its Achilles heel. The colon will become exhausted by reacting to the strong stimulation of the purge, and it often takes several days for the colon to recover. In these circumstances the intestine has been emptied—which was the purpose of the operation—but it no longer has the strength to eliminate the new food wastes it is receiving. They will begin collecting in the colon and retrigger constipation. Purges are therefore not a means for treating constipation. They have no rehabilitative effect on the colon and should only be used rarely and for the shortest possible period of time.

Generally speaking, purges are not recommended, but in the cases when they are truly necessary, here are two that are as a rule quite tolerable.

Lubricating Purge: Castor Oil

A plant of wet regions, the castor oil plant (*Ricinus communis*) produces seeds rich in oil with laxative or purgative properties, depending on the dose. Contrary to laxatives and purges that only act in the colon, castor oil goes to work when it enters the small intestine. Its unpleasant taste is no longer an obstacle, as it is now possible to buy deodorized castor oil.

Castor oil has a lubricating effect on the intestine, but it also takes action by vigorously stimulating intestinal peristalsis.

Take 2 to 3 teaspoons of castor oil or more (up to 6 maximum) in the morning on an empty stomach.

Saline Purge: The Bertholet Purge

Cited in his book on fasting, the purge developed by Dr. Bertholet (from Lausanne, Switzerland) is effective and well tolerated by the body.

Mix 40 to 55 grams of magnesium citrate and 10 to 15 grams of sodium sulfate in ½ liter of lukewarm water. Drink within 30 minutes. Its effects will make themselves known several hours later.

ENEMAS

Enemas consist of introducing water into the colon through the anus using an instrument for that purpose. Their effects are threefold.

- The water introduced into the colon permeates the hardened, dried stools; thus, their water content increases. The stools soften and become more or less liquid, depending on the amount of water used and the length of time it remains in the colon. The crusts that have formed on the walls of the intestines are dissolved and eaten away by the liquid. Because of the large quantities of water present, the stools are easily transported out of the body, as is the case with diarrhea.
- The weight of the stools, added to that of the volume of water that has been injected (which can range from ½ cup to several quarts), applies pressure on the walls of the colon and on the anal sphincter, which stimulates the peristaltic movements of the colon and the defecation reflexes.

- When a substantial amount of liquid and matter rapidly exit the intestines, it creates a void that sucks in the matter located higher up in the intestines.

Out of these three effects, it is the liquefaction of the stools that is the most important benefit of enemas. The quantity of water to be injected will vary from one enema to another, as I am now going to show. The first two are simple, and for that reason can be performed by the person alone at home. The third method requires sophisticated equipment and it is therefore necessary to visit a therapist to have it done.

The Rectal Douche

Rectal douches are called for when constipation is slight or intermittent.

The rectal douche is the mildest form of enema. The small amount of water used—from ½ to ⅔ cup—only fills the terminating part of the colon: the rectal ampulla.

The introduction of the water is performed by an enema bulb. The bulb consists of two parts—the bulb itself, which is made of rubber, and the cannula, which is made of plastic. This second piece is the part introduced into the anus to perform the enema.

The purpose of the rectal douche is to liquefy the stools, but more importantly to trigger the suction that follows the evacuation of the water. The water that is injected is, in fact, not held in but eliminated right away. This is only a small amount of water, but with the stools that are expelled at the same time, a void is created that sucks down the materials lodged higher up in the colon. They fall down into the rectal ampulla and are evacuated as well. Their elimination can be encouraged even more by a second rectal douche performed minutes after the first one.

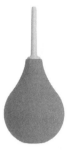

An enema bulb for
performing a rectal douche

The purpose of the rectal douche is to trigger the suction
movement that follows the evacuation of the water.

The rectal douche is a harmless procedure. Irritating effects
will be nonexistent provided the cannula is inserted gently and
carefully. If necessary, Vaseline or olive oil can be used to facilitate this maneuver. You must make certain that the bulb is full of
water in order to avoid injecting air into the colon. The temperature of the water used for this purpose should be close to that of
the body's temperature, so that it will be easily tolerated.

The rectal douche should be used daily, and if necessary for
several weeks in a row. This procedure will not make the intestine lazy. To the contrary, there is a stimulating and rehabilitative
effect on the peristaltic muscles and the rectal muscles that perform the actual evacuation.

Application

While standing upright, inject water into the anus with the help
of the enema bulb. Once the water has been injected, remove the
cannula and sit down on the toilet. The water is not held in, but
released immediately. The operation should be repeated two to
three times: the water that is expelled will be cleaner and clearer
after each procedure.

The 1-Quart Enema

Enemas using 1 liter or 1 quart of water are recommended when the constipation has become well established and the intestines are struggling to empty themselves.

This is the classic enema. The quantity of water injected will fill the rectal ampulla and a part of the descending colon. The water introduced into the body will be able to come back out quite easily. This is not the case with those enemas that use 2 to 3 quarts of water. Once the transverse colon and the ascending colon have been filled with water, the liquid will not flow as easily back out of the body.

The materials you will need for enemas can be found in pharmacies and drugstores. A complete enema tray contains:

- a graduated container for the water
- a long rubber hose
- a cannula equipped with a faucet

The purpose of the enema is to permeate the stools with water and thereby dissolve them. For this reason, the enema water is held in for several minutes before being expelled, so that it can remain in longer contact with the stools.

Bending the torso laterally will encourage the even distribution of the water and help it to blend with the stools.

One-quart enemas are recommended for one-time usage. A daily enema, repeated over a span of two or three days, is possible, but enemas should not be introduced with more frequency or for a longer period of time. Too-frequent use of enemas will exhaust the intestines and disrupt the intestinal flora.

The ideal temperature of the water should be in the neighborhood of 98.6 degrees Fahrenheit—the ideal human body temperature. Water that is too cold will trigger abdominal contractions; too hot and it will disagreeably heat up the colon or burn it. Tap water is perfectly suitable and can be used alone or with the addition of medicinal plant infusions. Depending on your needs you can use softening plants such as chamomile, stimulating plants such as alder buckthorn or coffee, or antibacterials such as eucalyptus or thyme.

Good to Know

The addition of 2 or 3 tablespoons of olive oil to the enema water will have a lubricating effect on the intestinal walls.

Application

The container should be full of water at the same temperature as the body. Place it higher than the rectum to allow the water to enter the intestines more easily. Insert the cannula in the anus with the faucet off. Kneel on all fours with the head and torso leaning forward, then open the faucet of the cannula.

You can facilitate irrigating the colon by breathing in deeply with the diaphragm or by slightly altering your position.

If the water pressure turns out to be too strong or painful, the faucet can be turned off for a minute or two.

You can also choose a prone position, lying down on your left side to facilitate the flow of the water toward the bottom of the sigmoidal loop.

Once all the water has been introduced into the colon, the cannula is removed. Hold the liquid in for a fairly long time (five to ten minutes) to ensure good liquefaction of the stools. Then, sitting on the toilet, empty the injected liquid and all the dissolved material it now carries.

Colonic Irrigations

This enema is the one in which the most substantial quantity of water is injected. In fact, during the first stage of this procedure, enough water is injected to not only fill the descending colon and the transverse colons, but the ascending colon as well. In the second stage, the water—now charged with dissolved material—flows out of the body but is immediately replaced by a flow of liquid running in the opposite direction. In this way a liquid transit is created that irrigates the entire colon.

The entrance and exit of the water is achieved thanks to a cannula with two circuits of tubes. A special apparatus is used to gently propel clean water into the colon through one of the cannula's circuit of tubes. When the colon is full, the second circuit of the cannula is opened, allowing the stool-charged water to leave the body. The supply of water through the colon remains continuous. As water leaves the body it is replaced by an equal amount of clean water—a current of liquid is thus entering and then leaving the colon. The presence of the water dissolves the hard stools as well as the material deposits coating the walls of the intestines. The stream of water has a scouring and corrosive effect on these deposits.

Two or three colonic irrigations will not only carry out a complete emptying of the colon but also a cleansing of the walls of the colon. An intestine cleaned in this fashion is ready to react effectively to the hygienic measures recommended in part 2 of this book. This procedure is primarily recommended for people who are severely constipated, but it is also beneficial for people who wish to cleanse their intestines.

The equipment needed to perform colonic irrigations is quite complex, so this therapeutic measure can only be carried out at the office of a therapist who is set up to provide this service. A cure of two or three colonic irrigations is generally sufficient but should be repeated two to three times a year for those people with especially sluggish intestines, or whose bodies are overburdened with toxins.

Table of Constipation Causes and Remedies

Causes	Remedies
Lack of roughage	Eat foods that are higher in fiber: fruits, vegetables, whole grains
	Take a high-fiber supplement: bran, psyllium, flaxseed
Lack of liquid	Drink 2.5 liters of water daily
	Take a hydrophilic supplement (one that draws water into the intestines): prunes, pears (dried), whey, lactose (milk) sugar
Hepatic insufficiency (sluggish liver)	Stimulate the work of liver with medicinal plants: artichoke, black radish, rosemary
	Hot-water bottle

Causes	Remedies
Consuming constipating foods or medications	Remove the foods at fault
	Eliminate the medications, if possible
	If not, compensate for their effects with a laxative
Lack of tone in the peristaltic and abdominal muscles	Exercises for the abdominal muscles
	Massages: kneading the intestines, tennis ball massage, massage of the reflex zones of the intestines
Imbalance of the intestinal flora	Strengthen the intestinal flora with prebiotics: foods high in fiber, whey, lactose (milk) sugar
	Reseed the intestines with probiotics: bifidus yogurt, active concentrates, laboratory products
Stress	Breath control
	Relaxation
Nutritional deficiencies	Fill the deficiencies through diet
	Take nutritional supplements: bee pollen, blackstrap molasses, brewer's yeast, seaweed

Illustration Credits

Drawings on pages 17, 106, 110, 113–20, 141, and 144 by Rosalie Vasey
Drawings on pages 22, 122, and 126, by Éditions Jouvence
Drawing on page 105 (bottom) by Stéphanie Roze

Photographs from Fotolia.com:

Page 3. © fresnel6

Page 4. © gpointstudio

Pages 10 and 12. © SenVietense

Page 24. © 7activestudio

Page 29. © Syda Productions

Page 31. © psdesign1

Page 35. © shaiith

Page 39. © monticellllo

Page 43. © Javier Castro

Page 46. © siraphol

Page 51. © Gina Sanders

Page 56. © Dionisvera

Page 59. © katrinshine

Page 65. © Mara Zemgaliete

Page 71. © Magdalena Kucova

Page 78. © ppi09

Page 81. © Meliha Gojak

Page 84. © nerthuz

Page 94. © Jürgen Fälchle

Page 99. © Brian Jackson

Page 105 (top). © ag visuell

Page 129. © leungchopan

Page 136. © Dušan Zidar

Page 146. © am

Page 154. © Grafvision

Page 157. © gattus

Page 159. © icarmen13

Page 168. © Comugnero Silvana

Page 172. © ILYA AKINSHIN

Index